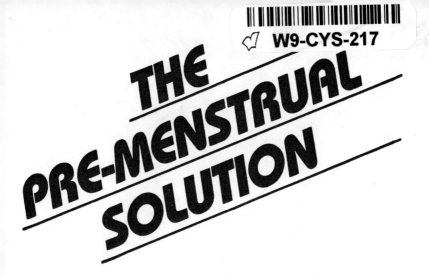

THE PRE-MENSTRUAL SOLUTION

HOW TO TAME THE SHREW IN YOU

by

JoAnn Cutler Friedrich, P.A.

Arrow Press, Inc.
1228 Lincoln Avenue, Suite 103
San Jose, California 95125
(408) 277-0976

Dedication

To my mother, with love and respect

Full Moon
(or PMS)

What is that indescribable tug
That surges within on the full moon?
Theories abound, surround and confuse
Adding to this disquieting mystery
Of my lunatical behavior

Whatever it is that seeps through
The caves of my helpless being
Is hidden in the deepest
Darkest oceans of my soul
Surfacing, timely
With that unfathomable tug

It rips at the tide within me
Until it froths and peaks
Forcing my emotions to charged pinnacles
Humbling thoughts and crushing humor
Riding the crests of never-ending, raging waves

I lust for unknown satisfaction
I lust for unknown revenge
I lust for unknown power
I lust, I lust, damn it . . .
For what do I lust?

It finally ebbs and crashes
What is left of me
Upon the jagged rocks of exhaustion
My emotions wallowing to and fro
Like sandy fragments of futile nothingness

Relieved . . . spent
Floating on calm waters
I seem uncaring and unaware of
The devastating impact on
My now impatient world

Yes, my wondering, accusing, thrashed-out world
Faced with the start of yet another cycle
Dreading the welling up, the rising tide
The unknown, lustful war within
That all-consuming, indescribable tug

Bonnie L. George

Contents

Acknowledgments

Michael Friedrich—*My husband and friend, your love and support through all the years of PMS turmoil sustained me. I appreciate you and all the sacrifices you made through the long months of research—I owe you many dinners!*

Jill Chase Friedrich—*My daughter, your constant love throughout the years enabled me to go on when I thought there was no hope. I love you dearly. I missed our time together during the long months of research. I owe you and Anthony LeMarca several hours of* private *telephone time!*

Dorothy Cutler O'Roke—*My mother and my number one supporter, you have always been there when I needed you. You washed wet sheets for years and never complained. You listened to my PMS rages and still loved me. Your constant love and support enabled me to do the work I have chosen. I would need to write another book to recount what I owe you!*

Cecily Cosby—*My research partner and my friend, we did it; we have made a difference for women with PMS. Thanks for being there to share my PMS horror stories. Our research and discovery was for me a "once-in-a-lifetime" shared experience. I could not have done it without you. I think we're probably even!*

Anthony Mangan—*My friend and biofeedback specialist, you taught me to listen to my intuitive voice, and it has proven to be an invaluable lesson. You have always been there to listen when I wanted to talk, and that has been frequently. I think I owe you and Cynthia several hours of silence!*

Introduction

Good News for Women

Until a year ago, I had been suffering from Premenstrual Syndrome all of my adult life, from the time I began menstruating at the age of 12. As I grew older, the symptoms became more severe and long-lasting. Later, I became a student of medicine, and at present I am a fully licensed Physician's Assistant with a practice of my own. Thus, it may seem ironic that it wasn't until I was in my early thirties that I started looking for some kind of medical solution to my problem.

Until then, like so many women raised in the fifties, I assumed this monthly torture was something *all* women went through; and certainly I didn't want to be the sort of person who went complaining to all her friends about a trivial inconvenience that was supposed to be a "natural female phenomenon." According to some ancient legends and myths, none of which were given any in-depth analyses over the years, women were put on this earth to suffer the pits of despair once a month in silence. Those were the dues they had to pay just for being one of the "weaker sex." What I didn't suspect, however, was that there were so many other women who were suffering as intensely as I, but who were equally reluctant to talk about it. Like me, they felt this was a very private matter, and, thus, the thought of turning it into a topic for conversation was, at the very least, in extremely bad taste.

The fact that I was part of the medical community while I was experiencing these symptoms might lead some people to think I would be more apt to find a solution than a layman. In my case, the opposite was true. I didn't really want to discuss this problem with anyone. Because of my professional standing I felt I should be able to control myself and chose to remain stoic and suffer in silence for many years, even though it was during this period that I was treating women patients for the same problem. I was doing a lot of listening and empathizing, but not much else. At the time, though I could certainly understand what they were going through, I could only commiserate with them. I didn't feel it would do too much for my credibility to let these patients know I was having the same problems but was powerless to solve them. After all, I was supposed to be invincible.

At this time, I was already familiar with most of the medical literature on the subject of PMS and had tried all the currently recommended programs, including all those over-the-counter placebos that do so little for so many. Consequently, I felt there wasn't anything out there that could make any difference. I was even more reluctant to discuss these symptoms with a doctor, and

I particularly did not want to talk about this with another Physician's Assistant since, like so many OB/GYN specialists, most PA's also happen to be men. And in my case, as I'm sure it must be for many women working in the professions, there was the fear that if I let my male competitors know about this problem, they would be quick to point out that I was operating in diminished capacity at least part of each month.

I have found that notwithstanding all their scientific enlightenment, many male specialists profess PMS to be a trivial problem caused by self-induced "hysteria," and that, as such, it would reoccur monthly, ultimately disappearing with the onset of menopause.

As for seeking the advice of a lady gynecologist, during those dark ages—and mind you, I'm talking here about the seventies and the early eighties—how could I be sure I wouldn't get another lady specialist who might be suffering in silence with this same problem, but, who, like me, had become programmed not to talk about it? The way my luck was running at the time, that could easily have happened.

In my case, although I suffered the usual somatic reactions as well as extreme fatigue, the most devastating symptoms were the emotional ones. I would have wild verbal rages, followed by frenzied fits of depression and sobbing. My husband and my daughter, in fact, were literally suffering from combat fatigue and were jumpier than I was when they knew I was about to start climbing the walls again. At my worst, they were probably a lot more conscious of the calendar than I was. I'd go into my Jekyll & Hyde routine, and in our house that was like a warning cry: "Alert the troops! Mom's riding her broomstick again!"

By the time I launched my desperate search for a real solution, my PMS symptoms were lasting about 14 days out of every month. Then there would be one week when I was having my period, and while that came as something of a relief after what I had suffered premenstrually, it still meant I was spending more than half my life in torment. I felt I would have to be some kind of hard-core masochist simply to lie down and let this go on destroying my life without putting up a fight.

That's where my friend, Cecily Cosby, entered the picture. She and I had been co-workers and good friends for many years. When we finally opened up to each other, we discovered we were both in the same premenstrual boat, which was sinking fast. It meant a great deal to me to have someone else with whom I could share this private horror. Knowing we both had a very personal reason for wanting to find a solution kept us strongly motivated for the long and painstaking period of research that lay ahead for us.

In the beginning, it wasn't as if we set out to do anything monumental in the way of an in-depth investigation. We simply meant to review all the existing literature we could find on this subject, and by doing so, we gradually found we were charting out areas which no one had bothered to investigate in the past. Our initial reasons were only to find a cure for ourselves. But when we finally struck gold—after more than two years of digging in the archives—the larger view took hold, and we began to see how many other women could be helped by the simple and inexpensive remedy we had literally stumbled upon. In short, the treatment program we will discuss in this book came to us by way of serendipity.

Much to our astonishment, the sure-fire tonic we discovered turns out to be a food supplement that can be obtained over-the-counter at any health food store. This means it is not classified as a drug by the FDA.

To end the suspense, what we're talking about is one of the 22 amino acids which help to augment a certain chemical in the brain known as serotonin, a process we will discuss in more detail later in this text. The amino acid we found effective is called l-tryptophan. When we used this remedy in a carefully prescribed manner which enables it to get into the brain, the improvement after only a few weeks was downright miraculous. Not only did this treatment prove effective for Cecily and myself, but now, after more than a year of treating hundreds of other Women, all have reported the same extraordinary results.

The question arises: Why didn't someone discover this simple solution sooner? The answer: Nobody cared enough to look. As for the male population, many laymen and doctors made it clear they were still sticking to their century-old gentlemen's agreement: There was only one "female condition" they cared to hear about, that of their ladies being in heat, rather than torment. And since most of us have steadfastly refused to talk about it, over the years we women have given them our fullest cooperation.

But now that this long, unhealthy silence has come to an end, a wholly new kind of feminist freedom will be possible for those of us who have been fighting a losing battle for so many years. The reason I wrote this book is to share this simple solution with the many other women who may be suffering these symptoms, but who have either been too ashamed or discouraged by the lapses of medical science to ask for help.

It is interesting to note here that in the past there have been countless books and surveys written on this general subject, and while most of them have been carefully researched and documented, whenever they made any specific reference to PMS, all they did was to explore and redefine this phenomenon. To my knowledge, *this is the first book on record to offer a real solution to the problem*.

We should also note that from now on, PMS need no longer be dismissed as if it were just another "Orphan Disease," the kind that is either too rare or too distasteful to warrant any costly research. On the contrary, the time has come to pay this worldwide malaise all the attention it has long deserved.

1

Fifteen Years of Borderline Insanity

How My Own PMS Nightmares Helped Show Me The Way

THE SPORTS WORLD RECOGNIZES the catch-phrase "no pain, no gain." As I look back I suspect that was the equation working for me. I suffered many years before I grew desperate enough to put an end to it. I knew in my heart that women were *not* put on this earth to suffer the tortures of the damned once a month, and I was determined to do everything in my power to put a stop to it.

I didn't really identify PMS as a problem until I was in my twenties. Before that, during adolescence, I didn't connect the fact that my fluctuating mood swings always occurred before my period. At such times, I would become testy or short-tempered, but most people attributed this to my being just another moody teenager. Or perhaps my mother would say, "Oh, you're just about to have your period," implying it was normal for me to be irritable at this time, and this was her way of welcoming me to the Sisterhood.

As it happened, my mother had also had a difficult time with PMS. However, she had been brought up in an era where nice people didn't discuss such things, which possibly explains why so many nice people grew up misinformed. As for my father, I'm sure it was his dismissive attitude about this subject that helped keep me quiet about the problem for so many years. He had some negative feelings about women having their periods and wouldn't permit other men to joke about it or even mention it in his presence. He gave me the feeling there was something mysterious and unmentionable about the whole process. I'm sure if someone had suggested that all women be quarantined during this time of month, my father would have been the first to agree. I suppose this attitude was fairly typical of men of his era, though I suspect it still holds true among some of today's die-hard chauvinists.

In any case, it was my father's attitude that further convinced me this wasn't the sort of thing for me and the girls to talk about after school. I also felt that if this were such a normal procedure for all females, what was there to talk about? Even when my symptoms worsened over the years, I still believed that all women suffered equally, so why fight the system? In high school, and even later, during college, I had never overheard young women discussing these problems in any great detail, except, perhaps, to briefly assure one another they had everything under control in that area. In fact, in those days it seemed we talked about everything else *but* PMS. Surprisingly, despite the permissive new attitudes of the mid-sixties, when everybody aired opinions about "the pill," sexual freedom, open marriage and wife-swapping, the subject about what happened to ladies at "that certain time of the month" was still taboo.

It was during my early twenties, after a failed first marriage and the birth of my daughter, Jill, that my PMS symptoms grew more intense and long-lasting. I'm sure this problem was at least instrumental in ending that marriage. Even before I was married, it had cost me several other relationships with men. In those moods of deep depression and melancholy, I didn't want anybody near me. Or if a boy friend happened to phone me at that time, I'd be in such a despairing, near-suicidal mood, I might say, "I never want to see you again. I can't stand the sight of you!"

It didn't occur to me to appeal to their humanity by saying, "I'm having my period now. Can you call back later?" I was afraid one of them might say, "But that's what you told me last week!" Rather than have any of those men know exactly how long these moods were lasting for me, I preferred to have them think I was rejecting them, not the other way around.

The enormous fatigue I always felt at this time was probably the most frustrating symptom for me, as there was so much I wanted to do with my life. It seemed I was always tired during those crucial weeks, and regardless of how many hours I slept, I would wake up feeling just as tired. Yet, despite that debilitating symptom, I managed to accomplish a tremendous amount of work over the years. "Being lazy" was not a natural choice for me. I went to school full-time, worked full-time and, until I married my present husband, I raised my daughter alone.

Fortunately, I was able to control these moods in a work-situation, but this involved such a studied and concentrated effort, I would really feel the repercussions when I got home at night, and so would my family. I suppose I didn't feel I had to impress anyone at home, so as soon as I swept through the door, I would let go with all the rage and bitchery I'd been holding back all day.

And yet, because I remained so controlled on the job, none of my business associates ever suspected I had this problem. I have since found out that many professional women suffering these symptoms are able to postpone the worst of it on the job. In my case, being around other people at work, plus the demands of the work itself, would serve as a kind of diversion therapy for me. But at home there was no reason for me to keep up the pretense.

During the years when I raised my daughter, Jill, alone, I'm sure she was both confused and frightened by my periodic rages and moods. I never abused her physically, but I know I did verbally. Simply because she was near me while I was feeling these symptoms, she would be the one I took it out on. I remember the times when I would fly into a rage over nothing at all; I would scream, kick her toys, and, from a little girl's standpoint, I must have sounded more like the Wicked Witch of the West than anybody's mother. Sometimes she would stare up at me, as if to ask, "Who *is* this crazy lady?" True, I would be aware of her feelings at such times, and it would worry me. But that worry was powerless to change these compulsive mood swings once they took over.

Nor would I ever want to apologize for my behavior

once my period was over, as that was the time when I preferred not to think about this problem at all. Somehow, I could even pretend that it had never happened and, even more incredible, that it would never happen again. No matter how faithfully this cycle returned each month, each time it faded away I would tell myself, "I'm not going to feel that way next time." And I truly believed this. I suppose the only explanation is that it's very easy to forget pain, and I must have wanted to forget so much that I was always ready to say "let the good times roll" whenever the bad times were gone . . . until they came again.

My present husband, Michael, to whom I've been married for ten years, let me know he was sensitive to these feelings, and there wasn't a doubt in my mind that he was truly concerned for me. But I'm afraid my knowing that didn't spare him. As with my daughter, simply because he was around when I experienced these symptoms, I would make him as miserable as I was.

Naturally it helped to know how perceptive and understanding he was, especially when he would advise me to . . . "Just be logical about it, honey. You know your period is due and that you'll have a bad time of it for awhile. But you also know it will pass." The poor darling, he was trying to appease me *before* I freaked out. But it never worked. Indeed, if he gave me that advice while I was already on one of my rolling rages, I might well respond by saying, "What the hell do *you* know about it?"

On the other hand, despite our inevitable fights at these times, and even though I knew he was powerless to help me with this problem, in a wistful sort of way I really did hope he could find some way to rescue me.

Part of my desperation at this time came from his inability to help me. I would think, "Michael, you're the most important person in my life, so why can't you make me feel better? If you really loved me you would lift me out of this."

I would also have other ambivalent feelings about my husband during these periods. For one thing, during the throes of PMS, I would long to have him come and hug me or comfort me, or even make love to me, a contradictory desire as it turned out, since at this time I couldn't stand to have anyone touch me. This meant that I would be sending him a lot of confusing signals, like, "I need you to hold me and comfort me, but please don't touch me." The poor guy, the only way he could fill both those requests was to throw me kisses from across the room. As it turned out, no matter how sincere his efforts, there was no right thing he could do for me to "make it better."

Even more ironic and frustrating, at this time my sexual drive would increase. Thus, it developed into the kind of Catch-22 situation that served only to intensify my feelings of rage and futility. Moreover, whatever I did during PMS was geared (hopefully) towards making me feel better. I was ready to try anything. I would eat more for that reason, quite willing to tolerate an unwanted weight-gain, if that would help. Or, despite my aversion to being touched at this time, I would occasionally force myself to have more sex, thinking maybe this highly rated panacea would ease my symptoms. At such times, I'm sure my husband wondered if I had only married him for medicinal purposes.

Unfortunately, such outlets as food or sex only served as a fleeting diversion for me rather than a cure. After reading much of the literature on PMS, I decided I should begin to take vitamins, start an exercise program and improve the quality of my diet. These things were of course very difficult to accomplish, as I was always exhausted and irritable. However, even with the positive changes I had managed to make in my lifestyle, there was no noticeable improvement in my PMS.

In time, it seemed that my whole life was revolving around destructive and negative feelings and what I could do to abate them. As a result my values and priorities were constantly subject to distortion, due to PMS.

The Pattern: Temporary Insanity Once A Month

Each month, I waited for the choreography of my fits and starts to alter its course, just to break the monotony. But that never happened. Once I knew those premenstrual symptoms were on the way, the whole process unfolded as relentlessly as night follows day. Aside from the fatigue, depression and irritability already mentioned, there would also be a whole repertoire of accompanying physical discomforts, so that during the times when I was so depressed I wanted to kill myself, I could derive some scant consolation by knowing it wasn't "all in the mind," after all. If it had been I couldn't possibly be suffering such things as constipation, weight-gain, diarrhea, backache, headache, bloating, as well as a lousy-all-over feeling—just about everything except the heartbreak of psoriasis.

Although it's true, as I've mentioned, that I never wanted to dwell on the bad times long enough to offer my family any formal apologies like many other women after I was over the worst of it, I did remember my obnoxious behavior enough to try and compensate for it with my family. But this led to another problem: since I only had about a week when I was "normal," I didn't have the luxury of postponing this conciliatory behavior for too many days. There was a kind of urgency for me to spread all my sweetness and light as quickly as possible. Chances were that if I waited too long, I would already be battling the furies again before I'd had the chance to be adorable.

In some marriages, this seesaw pattern could also give both children and husband greater leverage with the PMS victim during those periods, albeit brief, when they know she'll be easier to manipulate especially if they're feeling in the least vindictive about her recent imitation of a poltergeist. In that case they might want to take advantage of any compensating mood of warmth and compassion, as if to say, "Let's really *get* her for putting us through the wringer again." It's safe to say that for all members of the family, both the "before" and "after" periods of PMS are a little like walking on eggshells. You proceed at your own risk.

During my early thirties I had two late miscarriages, and it was from then on that my symptoms reached their all-time peak. At this time, the only relief I had was when the premenstrual symptoms eased up and my period itself, i.e., my menstrual flow, took over. That told me the worst was over and that after only another messy day or two, I could forget about this nightmare until the next time.

It was during those years after my miscarriages that my rages on the home front also reached a new behavioral high. At the time, it took only a trivial incident to set me off during my PMS. For example, one bright Sunday morning, I sent my daughter and husband out to get some fresh-squeezed orange juice for our breakfast. But because the store I had sent them to was closed, they had the "gall" to come home with two six packs of Minute Maid. Normally, this would not have been cause for me to administer on-the-spot capital punishment. But at that moment I was about six days into my PMS, so I launched into one of my wailing fits of overreaction.

"Canned orange juice?" I screamed at them. "What are you two trying to do to me? What is this, some kind of conspiracy, just to see how much torment poor old Mom can take?" Deliberately building the fury, I grabbed those cans of orange juice and emptied them down the sink, cursing like an old sea dog every step of the way. Then I got my coat and purse and raced towards the back door, yelling back at them, "I'm mad as hell, and I'm not going to take this anymore! Especially from my own flesh and blood." The fact that Michael was not a blood relative didn't deter me. I was on a roll.

I then dashed out of the house and drove all over town, searching for fresh-squeezed orange juice as if my life depended on it. I couldn't find any either, so naturally I returned home and sobbed in my room for hours. Whenever Michael or Jill had the guts to knock on my door with an offer of sympathy, I would roar, "Go away! I don't want to hear your apologies. I hate you both . . . !"

It was so out of proportion that after a few hours, I forgot what they had actually done to cause my rage; I simply kept brooding over it long enough to be more and more convinced that the people I loved most had betrayed me, which meant I was surrounded by enemies in my own home and, thus, had nowhere to turn. For the next day or so, I refused to speak to Michael and ignored my daughter.

And yet, in my brain I knew how absurd the reality of this situation was. It was as if I were telling my husband, "If you can't get me fresh-squeezed orange juice when I want it, we're through. I want a divorce."

Meanwhile, even during the height of this tantrum, the logical person I really was stood apart and watched this performance with dismay, my own inner voices saying, "Why are you doing this, Jo Ann? It's so crazy, and it's not even you. Stop and think. Be rational." But the fact that deep down, I *knew* I was behaving irrationally couldn't change anything. Once those moods had control of me, there was no way I could fight back. It was like looking at the scene of an oncoming accident, knowing what was about to happen, but powerless to take any action to prevent it.

Soon these moods began to affect not just my family, but others I had to deal with during the day. I don't mean at work; there I still retained control. I'm talking about store clerks, bank tellers, all those peripheral people I really tried to be nice to when I was in my right mind.

For example, once when I went into a dry cleaners to pick up a garment the clerk said she was sorry but it wasn't ready. Since I was in one of my demented states at the time, that was my cue to take center stage. "What do you *mean* that dress isn't ready? You *promised* me!" Without realizing it, I had raised my voice several octaves, causing everyone in the shop to turn and stare at me. And yet, though I dimly realized I didn't really want such an audience, I still kept shrieking. "What a disgraceful way to do business. I mean, really, what kind of a chicken outfit are you running here?" And more words to that flaky effect. Then I stomped out in a rage, while, I'm sure, those poor clerks must have concluded: "What a bitch! Either she's going through an early change or having a late period."

Normally, I might have those feelings anyway, but I would have managed to keep them a secret while being civil and polite. But under PMS, I was governed by a whole new set of rules, most of them spelling out anarchy. Once again it would make no difference that deep down I would know very well what a shrew I was being, for once it started, this process was unstoppable.

This situation had grown so terrible that just before Cecily and I began our research, I was actually looking forward to menopause, that time in every woman's life when Mother Nature tells her it's time to throw in the towel and cease firing. When that happened, it would end my premenstrual horrors forever. In case that day was too long in coming, and if I really thought it would help, I was ready to have a hysterectomy and have my ovaries removed.

Luckily, it was right about then that Cecily and I got together and decided to search for some alternative answers of our own. In our new roles as medical detectives, we continued our search without letup. Sometimes the two of us would get together and brainstorm for hours, searching for the one clue that had been overlooked by concerned scientists of the past. As it turned out, it would have taken us a lot longer to find such scientists than to track down the research.

During the course of our investigation, as you will observe in the next chapter, it seemed we first had to take a quantum leap forward in order to find the key to this puzzle. When you remember we're talking about a mystery that has lasted since the beginning of time, you'll realize that for a couple of pioneers we were very fast on our feet.

Somehow we knew we didn't have forever. Time was running out.

2

How We Found the Missing Link

The Key to the PMS Puzzle

IN THE BEGINNING, Cecily and I began looking at every piece of literature we could find on PMS. That was our first step. But in time, it was as if the whole project had a mind of its own, until eventually it began leading us instead of the other way around. Now that we had joined together to compare notes, we knew that our PMS symptoms were much more extreme than the average. I was also finding out that not all women suffered as we did; and yet, the vast numbers of them who did were just as much at a loss about it as I had always been.

Using ourselves as guinea-pigs, we also experimented with every therapy available in our search for a cure. I went on a diet and did some strenuous exercise. Aside from a much-needed weight loss, nothing else changed. We then tried diuretics, numerous multivitamin formulas, hypnosis; but nothing seemed to work, not even a sweet-sounding concoction called Evening Primrose. But for us all of these so-called "solutions" were a total washout.

We also experimented with tranquilizers and antidepressants, which so many physicians prescribe for PMS patients as an expedient approach to the problem. We found that both the MAO-inhibitors and the Tricyclics—the most common categories of antidepressants—often had severe side effects. These drugs must also be taken for quite awhile for them to become effective, and to us this did not seem satisfactory in solving what was, after all, a cyclic disturbance. Finally, we were so concerned about the side effects and had had little relief of symptoms, that we began to seek the solution elsewhere. We worried that the medication might prove harder to survive than the disease.

Taking tranquilizers disturbed us for other reasons. In cases of depression, these drugs seem to intensify the emotional symptoms, since they are, after all, classified as depressants. Not only that, in most cases, tranquilizers only postpone or camouflage the symptoms without alleviating the condition. For example, the most prominent symptom of depression is not caring about anything, having no incentive, being listless and withdrawn, a symptom most tranquilizers intensify.

Finally, after eliminating all the abovementioned possibilities, Cecily and I tried the hormone progesterone on ourselves for a period of about six months. After reading all of Dr. Katharina Dalton's books on PMS and progesterone we were convinced that this was the answer to our PMS prayers. We both began on 400 mg. natural progesterone suppositories two to three times per day. The first month after using the progesterone I noticed a slight improvement in physical symptoms such as breast tenderness and bloating. Cecily and I both noticed a little less rage, however, we felt somewhat like we were in a fog. Progesterone does act as a central nervous system tranquilizer, much like tranquilizers that are prescription. Unfortunately, the alarming problem came after the period began. We both noticed there appeared to be a shift in the symptom pattern while using progesterone. Now instead of having symptoms premenstrually, we had them during the period. It seemed as though we either paid now, or paid later. But pay we did.

Whether or not there had been a placebo effect the first month, or whether I had built up a resistance to it is uncertain. But when we both agreed we were feeling worse and not better on this treatment, Cecily and I agreed to stop taking it.

The progesterone represented our last effort. By then we had been buried in this research for a full year. We had, of course, chosen not to study the so-called psychosomatic symptoms, nor the archaic "it's-all-in-your-head" theory, though at the time we had no idea how soon we would reverse those convictions, nor for what special reasons. Meanwhile, before we discovered the common denominator, the many unquestioned somatic components to PMS made the theory that patients were only "imagining" these symptoms invalid. From our own experience, we knew for a fact that the attending emotional problems were both real *and* connected to the somatic symptoms.

In any case, after a year of study, we had not been

able to isolate any one central causative factor that might have been responsible for PMS.

Then, finally, the answer came to us almost overnight.

PMS A Sleep Disorder?

About this time I had another good friend and associate, a nurse named Vicky, who also had PMS and who had frequently joined Cecily and me in our discussions. Vicky and I had something else in common, however, an old secret locked away in our past which must have been too close for us to view with the same kind of clinical detachment we had used in our approach to the rest of our research.

In short, both Vicky and I had a history of childhood bedwetting. Somehow we knew this about each other; we must have let it slip in the process of some harmless girl talk that had nothing to do with our PMS research. Most women with this problem are about as eager to talk about it as those with PMS, since childhood bedwetting has always carried with it its own stigma. I myself had wet the bed nearly every night until I was twelve.

As you can see, that didn't give me much of an intermission between the end of one embarrassing trauma to the start of another, for it wasn't too long after I stopped wetting the bed that I began having my period. In very quick succession I graduated from one malady which "nice" people didn't talk about in mixed company to an ailment that was equally as taboo. More important, in the view of the general public, both these conditions were regarded as some vague sort of "emotional" weakness.

True, the current literature no longer supports the theory that bedwetting has emotional causes, though when I was a child this was still the prevailing opinion. It may also be interesting to note that I was an only child and there are certain cliché conclusions about the only child being spoiled, pampered, self-involved, hypersensitive, or just plain weird. I'm happy to report I didn't fall into any of those pat evaluations during childhood. My parents were always very supportive, and never made me feel isolated or special in any way. Nor did they give me the feeling there was anything "freakish" about my nightly bladder problems.

If anything, my mother had a very practical approach to this problem. She bought twin beds for my room so that I could alternate from one bed to the other. Whenever I drenched one bed, I would hop right into the dry one. This meant my mother was never obliged to do emergency laundry duty in the middle of the night. Certainly she never pressured me about wetting the bed and was very protective in keeping it a secret from others.

Despite her acceptance of my bedwetting, my mother's secrecy about this problem helped program me for keeping the secret of my severe PMS as an adult. In a way, my childhood served as a kind of apprenticeship for what was to come. At some level I felt that I must have been a little quirky or abnormal to have suffered from both of these curses.

Until a casual phone conversation with my friend, Vicky, one night, it had never occurred to me to connect PMS and bedwetting. This seems odd to me now, since I certainly couldn't deny that they both stemmed from the same anatomical source, the brain. Of course, bedwetting had none of the agonizing attending symptoms of PMS. In fact, for me there were certain times when those symptoms were at their worst that, if I'd had the choice, I would have gladly started wetting the bed again.

At any rate, Vicky and I were talking about one of our children staying overnight with a friend. In a half-joking sort of way, this reminded us both of how impossible that would have been for us when we were kids, due to our special problem.

"I guess that makes us both a couple of throwbacks," I kidded. "Most of today's kids seem to be properly housebroken."

"Don't be so sure of that," said Vicky. "That's probably what most people thought about us, too."

"Yes, that's probably true," I said. "And as long as nobody noticed how busy my mother kept our washing machine, my secret was safe."

Then we talked about how nice it would have been if she and I had known each other as kids. That way we could have stayed overnight together for our own pajama party without either of us suffering any embarrassment. As long as our mothers supplied the rubber sheets, we could have had a ball.

And yet, the more we talked about this subject, the less eager we were to continue joking about it. Gradually, we began to see some very serious connotations in the "coincidence" of our having suffered equally from PMS and childhood bedwetting. A few months before that conversation, I had made up my mind to search for a key symptom that might be the one pivotal connecting link for women with severe PMS. I felt if we could isolate something that Cecily, Vicky and I had in common, perhaps that would be the key we were seeking. I felt there had to be something in our history that would link us together. But until that phone conversation, it seemed we were all quite different. Cecily was thin, while I still had a weight problem. I exercised, they did not. I drank caffeine, they did not. Nothing coalesced.

But as Vicky and I talked that night, and grew more serious in our discussion of bedwetting, I finally said, "Maybe that's it, Vicky, the missing link that connects us all to PMS." At first we both tried to laugh it off, and I think Vicky said that was silly, and what possible connection could there be?

Then we both went silent for a moment. We weren't laughing anymore, and I was almost certain I could hear what she was thinking.

"What about Cecily?" Vicky asked.

"You mean, did *she* wet the bed as a kid?"

"Yes. Did she?"

"I don't know," I said.

"You mean, after all the years you've been friends, you've never even asked her?"

"Oh, come on," I said, "How many friends have *you* tried to lose lately by asking them a question like that?"

For a moment that started us laughing again. But not for long. "Okay, then hang up and call her," Vicky said. "Do it now."

It was a little late, but I did it anyway.

As soon as she said a very drowsy "Hello," I knew I had awakened her. "Cecily, before you say anything, just answer me one question. Did you wet the bed?"

"Not lately," Cecily mumbled. "Now come on, Jo Ann, what's this all about?"

"What do you mean, 'not lately'?" I demanded. "If not lately, then when?"

"When I was a kid, of course. I wet the bed until I was about 12."

Bingo! We were off and running.

Which means we had the ball, but we still had to figure out which direction to carry it to score a touchdown.

With this new information we began researching a totally new area, determined to find out exactly how the similarity in our backgrounds related to PMS. True, bedwetting was something we had done in our sleep, while conversely, when PMS really had us by the throat, normal sleep was out of the question: no matter how long we slept, it left us neither refreshed nor particularly energized the next morning.

Nevertheless, we had to believe that in some way, *sleep* was also a primary connection here.

Bedwetters Anonymous: The Club with No Members

At this time we each had a few women friends who suffered from PMS. Because we had already discussed these problems with them, we felt that a little more probing wouldn't offend them. We found out that all seven of these women had wet the bed as children. Now, certain we were not hallucinating, we were confident enough to start talking about taking some kind of bedwetters' poll, or perhaps doing a survey. We discarded the idea of placing personal ads in some of the women's magazines. We had our doubts about the kind of responses we'd get to an ad asking former female bedwetters who were now going through premenstrual hell once a month to get in touch with us. And besides, we had already drawn up an extensive mailing list while conducting our earlier research.

We then sent out about 3,000 questionnaires to women with PMS. We felt that now that the term "bedwetting" was no longer undercover, we could ask anybody just about anything. From the existing statistics on bedwetting, we already knew that if you're over the age of seven, you're somewhere near the age group wherein 1 to 5% wet the bed. Of those, it must be noted that 60% were boys, and we will discuss these masculine symptoms later in the text. Since we were talking about a very low percentage, we were then prompted to do our more specialized questionnaire. In that way we could compile the vital statistics regarding bedwetting among women with PMS.

There were 52 questions on the questionnaire. This included a variety of questions on social and medical history, lifestyle, and sleep patterns. One of the questions, as if it were almost incidental, had to do with childhood bedwetting. We also included special questions to rate their PMS symptoms, giving them a multiple choice, i.e., "Mild, moderate, severe or incapacitated." According to how they rated their symptoms, we put them into different categories, then examined the varying statistics.

Out of the 3,000, we found that 392 women responded to the questionnaire. Among these no one who suffered only a mild form of PMS had wet the bed as a child. In the "moderate" category, 7% had wet the bed. In the "severe" category, 28% had wet the bed, and in the "incapacitating" category, 39% had wet the bed past the age of seven. Of the total respondents, 19% were bedwetters. It was then that the proverbial light-bulb lit up over our heads, and we were convinced we had made a revolutionary discovery.

The severity of PMS symptoms increased with the number of women who had wet the bed as children. Or, if you will, the more problems they had with PMS, the more likely it was that they had been bedwetters. On the questionnaire, we also had some questions regarding premenstrual sleep patterns, and 98% of the women who responded mentioned they'd had a disturbance in their sleep patterns premenstrually. These women noticed the sleep disturbance only during PMS, not necessarily through the rest of their cycles. Some people reported having insomnia just prior to their periods, while others reported having problems with intermittent insomnia, meaning they would wake up several times during the night. This would last from ovulation until their period, after which they would be so totally exhausted, they would sleep a great deal, due to the build-up of fatigue.

We felt the information about these sleep disturbances was relevant. But it was the widespread bedwetting connection that proved to be our strongest common symptom. Nothing else seemed to correlate as effectively. For instance, there wasn't a strong correlation between the kinds of contraceptives the women used. We also looked into the causes of bedwetting, first ruling out those bedwetters who had bladder problems. It is now believed that those bedwetters with no urological abnormalities may be suffering from a problem in their sleep cycle. They appear to be spending too much time in Stage Four sleep, and insufficient time in Stage Five, or REM sleep, which we will discuss in more detail later in the text. As a result, they had difficulty awakening. And too, their sleep was so deep, they didn't consciously perceive the contractions they may have been having in their bladder, and thus had no conscious control over a full bladder.

Further statistics revealed that about 15% of boys and 10% of girls at the age of five are bedwetters. But by the age of nine, only 1–5% of all children remain bedwetters. The bedwetting generally ceases as the child gets older and spends less time asleep.

Suffice to say, bedwetting, or "nocturnal enuresis," remains one of society's unsolved problems. One theory suggests that the child is in such a deep sleep, nervous impulses go unheeded. This indicates some underlying central disorder with sleep. Efforts to lighten sleep with antidepressant medication have provided some relief though in time this treatment only proved to be moderately successful.

The trouble here is that bedwetting can often have many varied and complex ramifications. For example, periods of severe domestic conflicts could cause the child to become sufficiently anxious and disturbed to bring on enuresis during the night. It is precisely because the causes of this ailment are not clearly understood that the typical physician or general practitioner in treating this common childhood complaint will often feel uneasy about prescribing or diagnosing the condition. He may reject the problem by passing it off lightly.

Interestingly enough, during our later seminars conducted for PMS patients, a few of the women complained of having teenaged children who were still bedwetters. At our suggestion and after consulting with their physicians, these mothers started them on our l-tryptophan Treatment Program, and after only a few weeks, their children's bedwetting had stopped completely. This leads us to believe tryptophan will turn out to have multiple curative powers. Needless to say, more research needs to be done in this area.

In the following chapter we will point out how the brain chemical, serotonin, led to our investigation of the 22 amino acids which, in turn, brought us to our discovery of l-tryptophan.

The Premenstrual Solution Self-Evaluation

PMS
SYMPTOM LIST

This self-test is to help you determine how severe your PMS is. Please indicate whether your symptoms are (0) absent, (1) mild, (2) moderate, (3) severe, or (4) incapacitating.

Absence from work/school 0	1	2	3	4
Abuse—verbal or physical 0	1	2	3	4
Accident-prone 0	1	2	3	4
Acne 0	1	2	3	4
Aggression 0	1	2	3	4
Alcohol—decreased tolerance 0	1	2	3	4
Alcohol—increased consumption . 0	1	2	3	4
Allergies 0	1	2	3	4
Anger 0	1	2	3	4
Anxiety 0	1	2	3	4
Apathy 0	1	2	3	4
Appetite increase 0	1	2	3	4
Assault 0	1	2	3	4
Asthma 0	1	2	3	4
Avoidance of social activities 0	1	2	3	4
Backache 0	1	2	3	4
Binges 0	1	2	3	4
Bloating 0	1	2	3	4
Breasts—swollen or tender 0	1	2	3	4
Breathlessness or suffocation 0	1	2	3	4
Bruise easily 0	1	2	3	4
Circulatory problems 0	1	2	3	4
Cold sores 0	1	2	3	4
Confusion 0	1	2	3	4
Constipation 0	1	2	3	4

Cramps—dull ache 0	1	2	3	4
Cramps—sharp pain 0	1	2	3	4
Cravings for salt 0	1	2	3	4
Cravings for sweets 0	1	2	3	4
Crying 0	1	2	3	4
Depression 0	1	2	3	4
Diarrhea 0	1	2	3	4
Disorientation 0	1	2	3	4
Dizziness 0	1	2	3	4
Drug Abuse 0	1	2	3	4
Epileptic seizures 0	1	2	3	4
Excitability 0	1	2	3	4
Facial swelling 0	1	2	3	4
Fainting 0	1	2	3	4
Fatigue or lethargy 0	1	2	3	4
Feelings of suffocation 0	1	2	3	4
Guilt feelings 0	1	2	3	4
Headaches—migraine 0	1	2	3	4
Headaches—tension 0	1	2	3	4
Heart pounding or irregularity ... 0	1	2	3	4
Herpes flare-ups 0	1	2	3	4
Hypoglycemia 0	1	2	3	4
Increased energy 0	1	2	3	4
Increased need to sleep 0	1	2	3	4
Increased sensitivity to light 0	1	2	3	4
Increased sensitivity to sound 0	1	2	3	4
Indecision 0	1	2	3	4

Insomnia 0	1	2	3	4
Intentional self-injury 0	1	2	3	4
Irritability 0	1	2	3	4
Irrationality 0	1	2	3	4
Loneliness 0	1	2	3	4
Loss of control (or fear of) 0	1	2	3	4
Mood swings 0	1	2	3	4
Muscle stiffness 0	1	2	3	4
Panic attacks 0	1	2	3	4
Paranoia or suspicion 0	1	2	3	4
Poor judgment 0	1	2	3	4
Poor coordination 0	1	2	3	4
Poor concentration 0	1	2	3	4
Restlessness 0	1	2	3	4
Sex drive—increase or decrease .. 0	1	2	3	4
Shakiness 0	1	2	3	4
Sleep disturbance 0	1	2	3	4
Spotting 0	1	2	3	4
Suicidal thoughts 0	1	2	3	4
Swollen hands, feet, ankles 0	1	2	3	4
Tension 0	1	2	3	4
Urge to hit or throw 0	1	2	3	4
Weight gain 0	1	2	3	4
Withdrawal 0	1	2	3	4

Total your score and compare with the ratings be-low. This will help assess the presence/severity of your PMS symptoms. Remember this is a general guideline and there can be many variables.

If your total score is:

1 – 50

Your symptoms are mild and probably interfere minimally on your lifestyle— even minimal symptoms can be alleviated.

51 – 110

You probably have moderate symp-toms. This is the category into which most PMS sufferers fall. Most women in this category feel they are just a little more moody or sensitive around per-iod time and the medical community has offered little help—until now.

111 – 175

You have severe PMS. Your symptoms may be lasting for two weeks every month—your concentration is de-creased you're not sleeping well—you wonder if there's something seriously wrong with you. The Premenstrual So-lution can change your life.

> 176

You have incapacitating PMS. You of-ten feel that you're losing your mind. Your family and friends never know what to expect from one day to another—Start The Premenstrual Solu-tion Today! It really can change your PMS forever.

MENSTRUAL CHART
(circle dates of period)
⊠ *Mild* ◪ *Moderate* ■ *Severe*

MONTH: _____

DAY:	1	2	3	4	5	6	7	8	9	10
# of hours of sleep:										
Fatigue:										
Restless sleep:										
Insomnia:										
Forgetfulness:										
Mood Swings:										
Aggression/rage:										
Paranoia:										
Confusion:										
Despair:										
Crying:										
Decreased energy:										
Panic:										
Irritability:										
Depression:										
Difficulty coping:										
Increased sexual drive:										
Breast tenderness:										
Abdominal bloating:										
Water retention:										
Acne:										
Easy bruising:										
Constipation:										
Food cravings:										
Headaches (migraines):										
Increased episodes of Herpes:										
Seizure/asthma:										

11	12	13	14	15	16	17	18	19	20	21	22	23	24	25	26	27	28	29	30	31

3

How Serotonin Led Us to the Answer

Maybe It Is All in Our Heads, After All

AFTER RECEIVING SUCH SURPRISING RESULTS from our questionnaires, we began to research backwards. We had to find out in exactly what way our bedwetting statistics related to PMS. Initially, we were concerned mostly with the emotional symptoms, as we felt those would be more closely aligned to sleep problems. We then tried to determine what was "normal" sleep, and how certain of the antidepressants might work in treating sleep problems. We researched the chemicals affecting sleep, as well as studied the latest literature on how people were thought to sleep, including such patterns as hibernation and somnambulism.

It was during our research about sleep patterns that we came upon the term serotonin. This signalled a chain-reaction of discoveries. From the study of serotonin we were led to the amino acids, and from there, finally, it was just one quick step to l-tryptophan. At that point, something clicked for me and Cecily, and we felt unquestionably *right* about our research. Together, we had cooked up the perfect recipe for the only effective treatment for PMS ever discovered.

Feeling like latterday Madam Curies we whipped out the champagne and let the party begin. Not for long, of course; there was still too much to do.

On the one hand it seemed so amazing to us that someone smarter than we, brandishing several doctoral degrees, hadn't put all this together long ago. On the other hand we surmised that this problem had never been considered "big" enough for the geniuses to tackle. What top scientist could hope for much fame or glory in researching an ailment that lacked public exposure and popularity? PMS was not the stuff of which Nobel prizes were won.

What Is Serotonin?

Serotonin is a chemical that is present in both your brain and your body's circulating system, and this holds true for both men and women. It must be noted, however, that the circulating serotonin does not pass into the brain, nor does the brain's serotonin pass into the circulatory system. These two separate systems of serotonin are not interchangeable. One is neuroserotonin, or brain serotonin, while the other is circulating serotonin.

So why is serotonin important to PMS? The answer is both simple and complex. To begin with and of significant importance, serotonin is a multitalented chemical that can be linked to all the symptoms of PMS. In the brain serotonin controls the quality of sleep. It is important in the regulation of appetite, and it is a critical factor in controlling when a woman ovulates in her menstrual cycle. It is also a neurotransmitter, in other words it is necessary to transmit messages from one part of the brain to another. Thus, it serves as a kind of messenger. If you don't have enough serotonin, the messages don't get through as rapidly. I know I often felt that I was "in a fog" premenstrually, and although I could continue to function there was a definite difference in my mental clarity before and after my period.

In the circulating system serotonin also plays an important part in premenstrual symptoms. Serotonin is important in our clotting mechanism; low levels may cause easy bruising. It is a vasoconstrictor, an important factor in migraine headaches, as they are caused from vasodilitation. Serotonin is also in the gastro-intestinal tract and may be important in the regulation of such symptons as nausea, vomiting, diarrhea and constipation. As you can see serotonin has varied and necessary functions in both the body and the brain. Each of these functions and their relationship to PMS will be described more completely later in this text.

Serotonin is produced every day by an amino acid called l-tryptophan (see Chart, pp. 41 and 42). L-tryptophan is an essential amino acid. This means it can be found in protein or other foods. When you ingest protein, you also ingest amino acids in combinations, of which tryptophan is only one. When you ingest the protein, it breaks down into the amino acids which then circulate into the system. Some of the tryptophan is pulled into the blood stream, causing serotonin to circulate. Some of the tryptophan is pushed into the brain, and that produces serotonin in the brain; and thus, we have two separate systems.

Exactly What Are Amino Acids?

Amino acids are the building blocks of our foods. Food is judged nutritionally on its content of amino acids. There are 22 amino acids and of these our bodies have the ability to make all but nine. Of course, it's critical that we have all the other ingredients to make the other 13, but nine must be obtained from the diet. Without these amino acids, human life cannot survive; hence, their presence in the diet is mandatory. Amino acids are the precursors to certain essential chemicals in our bodies. In other words if these amino acids are not present in our bodies, the chemicals our bodies require will be lacking. As you can see, we really are what we eat.

The Further Functions of l-Tryptophan

Tryptophan is among those essential amino acids that must be replaced daily in the diet, as the body doesn't have the ability to store it. This also means that the serotonin must be replaced daily in the body. Aside from being involved in our sleep cycle, our reproductive cycle, and our dietary patterns, serotonin is an important factor in relation to depression and certain behavioral changes, as well as influencing a variety of physical symptoms. Often referred to as the biogenic amine, serotonin acts both centrally and peripherally. The central effects include modification of hypothalmic-anterior pituitary functions. In the periphery it is found in platelets, where it helps with our bloodclotting mechanism. It is because it is so rapidly turned over in the body that it requires almost daily replacement.

Some of the factors that influence the synthesis and the metabolism of serotonin are diet, liver function and the general availability of tryptophan. Although it is, as we have discovered, a neurotransmitter, serotonin does not cross the blood brain barrier, but is converted from tryptophan once it has entered the brain with a carrier molecule. Because of serotonin's strong link to emotional and social behavior, it has a significant bearing in the treatment of depression, and is also why some antidepressants prove effective by increasing the serotonin. Because of the difficulty in measuring levels of brain serotonin, medical practitioners must experiment with different dosages of antidepressant medications until an individualized dosage is established.

It is also interesting to note that in the past few years medical researchers have regarded sleep as a possible cause of depression. It was generally believed that disturbed sleep patterns were symptoms of depression. But now I wonder if it isn't the other way around; perhaps the disturbed sleep patterns come first and then create the depression. I am referring to the amount of REM sleep when I say it's the quality of the sleep that matters most.

Laboratory tests have proven that if you deprive someone of sleep over a long period of time, they can become psychotic. This further indicates that the above-mentioned reversal might well be what is happening.

A key element in the biochemical theory of some

psychoses may relate to the amount of serotonin in the brain. Serotonin inhibits luteinizing hormone, as well as acting as a precursor to melatonin. In addition, serotonin either stimulates or inhibits a variety of smooth muscles and nerves, causing responses in the cardiovascular, respiratory and gastro-intestinal systems. When serotonin deprivation occurs in laboratory animals, there appears to be an association with affective disorders, suppression of REM during sleep, and an increase in sexual activity.

Other monoamines important to normal brain function include dopamine and norepinephrine. Their interaction is complicated. Alteration of physiologic activities is affected not only by synthesis, but also by storage, release, metabolism and excretion.

Basically, we found that serotonin is the one factor in PMS that links all the symptoms together. See Chart 30D.

How Serotonin Relates to PMS Symptoms

The major symptoms of PMS are as follows: fatigue, restless sleep, insomnia, forgetfulness, mood swings, aggression, rage, paranoia, confusion, despair, crying, decreased energy, panic, irritability, depression, difficulty coping, increased sexual drive, possibly increased episodes of herpes simplex, seizures, asthma, and migraine headaches.

We feel these symptoms relate to serotonin for the following reasons: as a neurotransmitter, serotonin is linked to behavior and mood changes. It is also necessary for conversion to melatonin and normal sleep. Lack

Symptoms

PMS SYMPTOM	RELATIONSHIP TO SEROTONIN

Fatigue
Restless Sleep
Insomnia
Forgetfulness
Mood Swings
Aggression/Rage
Paranoia
Confusion
Despair
Crying
Decreased energy
Panic
Irritability
Depression
Difficulty coping
Increased sexual drive
Possible increased episodes
  of: herpes, seizure,
  asthma, migraine
	Serotonin is:
	• a neurotransmitter linked to behavior and mood changes.
	• necessary for conversion to melatonin and normal sleep. Lack causes sleep deprivation symptoms.

Breast tenderness Abdominal bloating Water retention Acne	Serotonin inhibits luteinizing hormone. Uninhibited LH may cause early ovulation and a shift in normal estrogen and progesterone during the luteal phase.
Easy bruising	Serotonin promotes platelet aggregation.
Constipation	Serotonin found in GI system.
Food cravings	Low levels of brain serotonin causes carbohydrate cravings.
Headaches *(migraine)*	Serotonin is a powerful vaso-constrictor.

of Stage 5-REM sleep can also cause these symptoms. For example, patients with a history of asthma, migraine or seizures are more apt to have episodes of these illnesses after they have been sleep-deprived.

In its role as a neurotransmitter, serotonin helps transmit messages from one part of the brain to the other. Low levels of brain serotonin may cause a delay in the messages getting through rapidly, causing a feeling of mental confusion, and a lack of general mental clarity.

A second set of symptoms in which serotonin plays an important role includes what I call physical symptoms, such as breast tenderness, abdominal bloating, water retention and acne. Because serotonin is critical to the timing of ovulation, low levels may cause early ovulation and a shift in estrogen/progesterone patterns. This shift in the normal estrogen/progesterone patterns can cause the above mentioned symptoms. This will be discussed in more detail later in the text.

Another PMS symptom is easy bruising, and since we know that serotonin promotes platelet aggregation and is important in the clotting mechanism, this means it could prevent this symptom, while, if you are low in serotonin, chances are that you will bruise more easily.

Serotonin is also helpful in the treatment of migraine headaches because sleep deprivation can intensify these headaches. But with migraine headaches, there is also vaso-dilitation, which means that the vessels are dilating. Since serotonin is also a powerful vaso-constrictor, it can help to abolish these symptoms.

We have found that serotonin is also instrumental in controlling constipation, nausea and diarrhea, which, in other words, makes it an incredible cure-all. The universal impact of serotonin really takes it out of the specialized realm of PMS, for these identical brain chemicals also control the symptoms of so many other ailments, which are suffered by men as well as women. For the same reason, the food supplement, tryptophan, is also being recommended as a treatment for sufferers of migraines, chronic headaches, lower back pain, and arthritis. Like bedwetting, it appears to affect a long list of ailments which we previously assumed we had to accept as a normal way of life.

Metabolic Pathway of Tryptophan

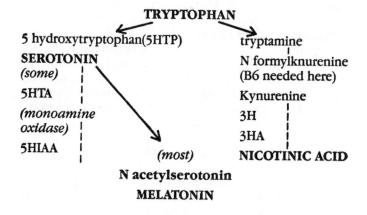

TRYPTOPHAN

5 hydroxytryptophan(5HTP)

SEROTONIN
(some)

5HTA

(monoamine oxidase)

5HIAA

(most)

N acetylserotonin

MELATONIN

tryptamine

N formylknurenine
(B6 needed here)

Kynurenine

3H

3HA

NICOTINIC ACID

Tryptophan:

One of nine essential amino acids. Crosses the blood-brain barrier with a carrier protein that insulates it from insulin. Competes with other amino acids to cross the blood-brain barrier. Must be replaced daily in the diet; scarce in food proteins. Precursor of Niacin (60 mg tryptophan-1 mg Nicotinic Acid). Low B6 can alter its metabolism. Converted to serotonin, then melatonin for sleep.

Serotonin:

Stress causes increased uptake and metabolism. Neuroserotonin converted from tryptophan. Blood serotonin found in plasma and platelets. Rapid turnover; must be replenished daily. Biogenic monoamine. Influences sleep mechanism in the brainstem; required for NREM and REM sleep. Decreased uptake with MAO inhibitors causes more to be available for sleep. Powerful vasoconstrictor. Converted to melatonin in the Pineal gland. Important for platelet aggregation and the control of the secretion of prolactin. Key element in the biochemical theory of some psychoses.

Melatonin:

Modifies behavior and EEG activity. Production triggered by hypothalmus, detection of SCN (suprachiasmic nuclei). Inhibitory effect on gonadal and thyroid function. Suppresses secretion of pituitary luteinizing hormone. Influences normal sexual maturation. Production signaled by light-dark change and the optic nerve. Enhances secretion of prolactin. Necessary for sleep.

Nicotinic Acid:

Two forms exist. Niacin (nicotinic acid) is easily converted to its amide form, nicotinamide, which is water soluble and stable to acid and heat. It is a partner with riboflavin in the cellular coenzyme that converts proteins and fats to glucose and that oxidize glucose to release controlled energy. Clinical manifestations of riboflavin or niacin deficiency are closely parallel, and if one of these two components is deficient, the other is usually deficient as well. Minimum required for necessary tissue stores is about 9 mg/1000 calories. Meat is a major source, also peanuts, beans, and peas. Diseases associated with niacin deficiency include pellagra, the greatest prevalence being in women ages 20-45 (the childbearing, lactating group). Diet alone can cure, prevent, or cause the disease. Pellagra causes among other symptoms general nervousness, confusion, depression, insomnia, apathy and delirium (similar to those of partial sleep deprivation). Either a deficiency in dietary tryptophan or nicotinic acid causes this disease, and it can be treated with either. Mental symptoms generally clear after treatment of three to four days. (Partial sleep deprivation symptoms generally clear in three days.)

4

Sleep and Its Importance to PMS

Dreams, the Stuff That Sleep Is Made Of

NATURALLY, we all feel at our best when we get what we perceive to be a normal night's sleep. Some of us may get by with less sleep, while others will require more than the average amount. But we all know that going without sleep for an indefinite period of time can create a variety of debilitating symptoms.

When we refer to "adequate" sleep, we are taking into account both the length and the quality of the sleep. This is a must for people who want to wake up feeling both mentally and physically refreshed.

There are five distinct stages of sleep. Stages One through Four consist of non-REM sleep, while Stage Five sleep is called REM (rapid eye movement) sleep, the stage in which we dream. Generally we pass through all five stages of sleep in approximately 70 minutes, and then repeat that cycle about six times during the average night.

Current statistics indicate that women require about an hour more of sleep than do men. However, I have come to believe after working with hundreds of women with PMS, that they require even more than this one extra hour of sleep, particularly during their premenstrual periods. Due to the poor quality of sleep they've had, women in the throes of PMS often wake up from a night's sleep feeling more tired than when they went to bed. This can be the case even if they have slept as long as 12 hours.

There are two alternating physiological sleep mechanisms for non-REM and REM sleep, and they both lie in the brain stem and are both influenced by serotonin. The destruction or suppression of serotoninergic neurons results in insomnia and thus a disappearance of both REM and non-REM sleep.

To be more specific, we experience two different changed states of consciousness during the night and pass through five distinct stages of sleep. The quiet non-REM consciousness state is Stage One. A light beginning sleep in which we drift through Alpha into the Theta brain wave range is Stage Two. A moderately deeper state of Theta brain wave activity is Stage Three, while a deeper state of slow Delta brain wave activity is Stage Four, the deepest state of Delta sleep. The active REM consciousness state is Stage Five, REM sleep. This is a light dreaming state of sleep during which brain wave activity increases.

A sleeper may actually spend approximately 20 minutes actively dreaming during Stage Five. At this point the cycle ends and the sleeper enters Stage Two of the following sleep cycle. Thus, you go through Stages One, Two, Three, Four then back up to Three then to

Two before you can enter Stage Five. When the dreaming Stage Five ends, you then go back into Stage Two sleep and repeat this cycle.

During sleep, the body rests. But the brain goes through approximately five very active periods of dreaming each night. Sleep has been described as an overnight battery charge for the body. Both bone formation and body growth accelerate during sleep, but cell rejuvenation actually goes on 24 hours a day. Therefore, we don't feel that sleep is biologically necessary for body restoration, but that it originated as a survival habit during evolution, and that the mental processes of learning perception increased during sleep.

The Stuff of Dreams

In many aspects, our dreams tell us how we should act though most nightly fantasies appear to be telling us how we should cope with the many changes of life. Studies have shown that, in fact, dream material is presented in a distinctly fixed order. During the night our minds scan up and down processing information and putting it together in new combinations.

During the first dream of the night the mind presents an overview of what problems it wishes to solve. The second and third sleep cycles during the night integrate the present problem with similar problems in the past and feelings about these past events. The fourth sleep cycle is concerned with making decisions about problems and events we face in the future. The fifth dream cycle consolidates information from the previous cycles and presents a final dream that is symbolic in nature.

If, in fact, dreaming is a time set aside to problem solve and make decisions that are important to our lives, then it would seem most dreams would be concerned with stressful events. In research done at the Dream Research Institute it was shown that negative emotions are involved in most dreams (75%). They further found that 50% of all dreams concern misfortune, while 33% concern things we fear or are anxious about.

Consequently, all dreams are built around problems or failures, while few, if any, concern success or good fortune. Without REM periods of sleep, I feel it would be virtually impossible to cope with the stresses of life. In a sense, dreams offer a preview of upcoming anxieties and the skills necessary to handle them.

Many sleep researchers who specialize in dreams believe that the emotions we express in our dreams prepare us for future events such as childbirth, job interviews, college exams, and so forth. Dreams may, in fact, give us the skills we need to cope with these stresses. For example, a study done on pregnant women showed that those women whose dreams embodied fear and anxiety spent less time in labor. Other studies have confirmed that those people who are about to face a traumatic life event spend more time in REM sleep. Psychologist David P. Cohen at the University of Texas Sleep Laboratory found that volunteers who were subjected to an ego-threatening experience prior to sleep and who then spent time dreaming about that experience were less tense than those who did not dream about the same experience.

There is a great deal of evidence to suggest that dreams are a psychological release during which the right hemisphere of the brain deals with suppressed anxiety, rage, and hostility. For instance, the more problems we face or the more learning we do, the more time we spend in REM sleep. As a matter of fact, REM sleep actually increases after any form of stress, learning or anxiety. When people are deprived of REM sleep, their learning ability declines and they are less able to cope with emotional problems.

Other studies show that both animals and humans become restless and irritable when they are deprived of REM sleep. When allowed to sleep naturally once more, both experience REM-rebound, which means they will compensate by spending long hours in dreaming. When a person is awakened before reaching REM, he will go through Stages One through Four faster during the next sleep period than would normally be expected.

Moreover, without REM sleep, we have difficulty in assimilating the stressful experiences of the day. Numerous studies have also linked REM sleep with learning ability. Other researchers found that when sleepers were shown a series of everyday objects and asked to memorize them, those who spent the greatest amount of time dreaming had the best memory recall.

The Pineal Gland and Melatonin

The regulation of sleep takes place in a part of the brain called the pineal gland, which is an obscure organ that is buried near the center of the brain. Named because of its resemblance to a pinecone, the human pineal is smaller and weighs less than an aspirin. Its existence was chronicled by the early Greek anatomists, but there have been sharp disagreements over its function ever since the fourth century B.C., when Herophilus suggested that the pineal was the "sphincter of thought," the mind's valve. Rene Descartes, the 17th century French philosopher, went him one better when he called the gland "the seat of the rational soul."

It is in the pineal that the hormone melatonin is manufactured throughout each night. It is this hormone that induces people to become sleepy and experience both REM and non-REM sleep. It is something of a miracle the way melatonin works on the sleep mechanism.

Here's what happens when you feel you're about to "drop off" for the night:

During the daytime, when the eye (optic nerve) is perceiving daylight, your brain stores serotonin for later use in your sleep cycle. But when your optic nerve perceives darkness, the serotonin is rapidly converted into the chemical melatonin. During the day, light inhibits melatonin production in the pineal. But the gland is not idle. From dawn to dusk it converts the amino acid tryptophan into serotonin, the substance that will be turned into melatonin at night.

The melatonin is acted upon by other chemicals, an enzyme called Acetyltransferase, or NAT, which rises dramatically each night, and Hydroxyindole-D-Methyltransferase, or HIOMT, which also increases, but less dramatically. Thus, in a two-step process, serotonin is changed into melatonin and released into the bloodstream, which first causes drowsiness, then sleep. With the onset of darkness, the neurotransmitter norepinephrine is released by nerve cells connected to the pineal and triggers the hormone factory. This entire process is activated by the way your eyes perceive light and dark.

When you awaken in the morning, and your eyes perceive light, the melatonin is rapidly converted back into serotonin. This causes me to wonder about the inevitable changes that must have taken place since the time when our ancestors went to sleep when the sun went down and rose when the sun came up. This was long before electricity gave us the kind of control over our sleeping habits that we enjoy today. Now that we have shuffled these patterns around, I wonder if that hasn't helped contribute more problems in relation to PMS.

Sleep Deprivation

Sleep deprivation falls into two categories—total sleep deprivation, wherein one is deprived of all manner of sleep from sixty to two hundred hours, or partial sleep deprivation, wherein one is deprived of REM sleep chronically over a period of several nights.

Total sleep deprivation of both NREM and REM sleep can cause any or all of the following symptoms: fatigue, irritability, decreased concentration, inaccurate perception, disorientation, deterioration of motor task performance, depression and hallucination. In certain predisposed individuals, it may also provoke psychotic episodes with bouts of screaming, sobbing, incoherent speech, delusions, and paranoia.

Most people who have been deprived of sleep will find it easy to relate to these symptoms. They experience everything almost second-hand, from a hazy distance, or as if they are moving through life underwater. It's interesting to note here that women going through PMS describe exactly that feeling, even after they have slept without interruption all night long. It can possibly be equated with the disoriented feelings caused by jet lag: the feeling that you are not really where you're supposed to be, though you know perfectly well that you are. You are simply perceiving the familiar in a different way, because now the familiar is unreal. These are similar to the feelings we get when we are deprived of normal sleep for a long time.

There is also the possibility that my tryptophan treatment might work with jet lag. With jet lag you alter the hours of your sleep, which takes you off your interior clock, or the circadian rhythm, controlled by the pineal gland. It seems that you can alter this clock an hour or two earlier or later without causing too much disorientation, but when it is a matter of from five to eight hours time difference, it may take several weeks to readjust. This is the result not only of the lack of neurotransmission, wherein the serotonin transmits the message from one part of the brain to another, but also of normal sleep deprivation.

These symptoms also bring to mind a recent psychiatric study that was done with a group of people living in Portland, Oregon. Instead of jet lag or sleep deprivation, these people suffered from a rare form of depression called Seasonal Affective Disorder, or SAD. More simply, this could also be called the "winter blues" because it starts soon after the Christmas holidays, and is especially prevalent in climates enshrouded in long months of grey and overcast weather. This form of depression is so debilitating that patients will often suspend all manner of activity or career involvement for four or five months at a time.

After a great deal of study, it was decided to experiment with these patients by having them sit close to a large panel of bright klieg lights, like those found on a movie set. This was done every morning and evening through the fall and winter. In time this Hollywood treatment nudged these people out of their winter doldrums into a psychological spring. While it's true that more daylight is definitely advised for many severe forms of depression, this sort of phenomenon could be happening elsewhere, though to a lesser degree. In many homes, there isn't a sharp enough light-and-dark contrast when converting serotonin to melatonin at night. This may well be what's happening to people who watch TV in a dim light for several hours before going to bed. There isn't that vivid changeover from light to dark. This could result in quite a delay before these people fall asleep.

Consequently, I wondered if the invention of artificial light during the Industrial Revolution might also be partly responsible for tampering with man's normal sleep patterns and rhythms. In a recent study done on depression, it was discovered that if people moved their sleep time forward several hours, and got up earlier, or if they went to bed at seven and got up at four in the morning, their depression disappeared. *In each of these studies, the symptoms are strikingly similar to those experienced by most women who suffer from PMS, and, when compared to conditions involving sleep deprivation, the symptoms are almost identical.*

How to Reverse the Damage Done by Total Sleep Deprivation

The good news here is that the amount of sleep required to recover from this long sleepless period never equals the amount of sleep lost. This means that if you've been deprived of sleep for 200 hours, it won't take you another 200 hours to catch up. In normal circumstances, however, it's never very healthy to alternate your sleep habits from one night to the next.

Initially, here is what happens to the person who has been deprived of sleep and then begins to sleep again: First, he falls rapidly into Stage Four or NREM sleep at the expense of the earlier stages. In a sense, this is because he is much too exhausted to bother with anything but very deep sleep. His sleep is then periodically interrupted with REM sleep in normally occurring amounts.

That was his first night of sleep after deprivation.

On the second night of sleep, Stage Five REM sleep rebounds, and it actually exceeds the amount of the pre-deprivation stage. Thus, the person manages to catch up on REM sleep during the second night, which means it takes about two or three days to catch up after total sleep deprivation. He begins to feel progressively better after the second and third nights.

Here we see another parallel with the symptoms women must tolerate during PMS, as they also claim that it takes a couple of days after the end of their cycle before they start feeling better.

Partial Sleep Deprivation

People who are prevented from REM sleep night after night exhibit numerous symptoms. They have a greater tendency to become hyperactive and are emotionally labile (vulnerable, combustible), which is probably the most prevalent state in which most PMS patients find themselves: they are ready to explode.

In this super-susceptible mood, women will repeatedly overreact to some trivial occurrence which serves as a surrogate target for their anger; what's really troubling them is the PMS state they are in, not whether or not somebody forgot to take out the garbage.

Partial sleep deprivation also corresponds well to the increased activity, excessive appetite and heightened sexuality of REM-deprived animals. Similarly, PMS patients will have more intensified emotional responses, as the symptoms of sleep deprivation—albeit chemically simulated—will tend to lower their resistance in general.

Categories of Sleep Disorders

Sleep disorders include insomnia, narcolepsy, nightmares, somnambulism (sleep-walking), and cataplexy, which is a sudden, temporary loss of muscle tone that renders the patient catatonic. As I discussed earlier, nocturnal enuresis (bedwetting) is also classified as a sleep disorder, except for those people who suffer from urological abnormalities. And according to my theory, PMS can also be categorized, at least partially, as a sleep disorder.

In order to normalize sleep habits, efforts should really be aimed towards increasing the amount of melatonin available as well as providing sufficient time for sleep. This process is two-fold: you increase NREM and REM sleep by increasing the melatonin, and you also increase the amount of time you sleep.

One last word of caution. It's best to find out both the quality and the quantity of sleep that works best for *you*. Then try to adhere to that pattern on a regular basis.

SLEEP IS THE KEY to eliminating the emotional symptoms of PMS. It's critical to the control of your PMS symptoms that you develop good sleep habits. Here to help you are some sleep do's and don't's.

SLEEP DO's

Do be consistent about taking your l-tryptophan and vitamins as outlined in this book.

Do develop regular sleep habits and stick with them.

Do sleep a minimum of 8 hours per night.

Do sleep in a dark, quiet and cool room.

Do sleep on a comfortable, firm mattress.

Do make your sleep time a high priority in your life.

Do discuss the importance of your sleep with other family members.

Do minimize sleep interruptions.

Do take naps if you are unable to get a full 8 hours sleep or have PMS symptoms.

Do increase your sleep just prior to ovulation to 9+ hours per night.

Do eat a well balanced diet.

Do exercise in the afternoon if possible.

Do consider sleep the most important factor in eliminating the emotional symptoms of PMS.

Do unwind prior to trying to sleep with an activity such as reading, TV or a hot bath—something you find relaxing.

Do some form of regular stress reduction.

Do give yourself permission to make time for yourself before sleeping.

Do make your room light upon arising by turning on
lights and opening drapes.

Do wash your face or shower upon arising to help you
wake up.

DO HAVE A GOOD NIGHT'S SLEEP, YOU DESERVE IT!

SLEEP DON'T's

Don't alter your sleep time more than one hour early
or two hours later than your usual bed time.

Don't eat a large meal high in protein prior to bed time.

Don't take sleep medications, tranquilizers or antihistamines to help you sleep.

Don't exercise just prior to bedtime or in the evening.

Don't try to sleep until you have taken time to unwind.

Don't drink large amounts of alcohol, an occasional
drink is OK (Moderation is the key here).

Don't drink large amounts of coffee or cola drinks
prior to bed (Again, moderation is the key).

Don't worry about falling asleep. When you have adequate amounts of serotonin and have developed
good sleeping habits, sleep will happen naturally.

Don't smoke (if your PMS is so severe you can't consider quitting now, then avoid smoking before
bed or during the night—you can quit later
when your PMS is in control).

Don't use artificial sweeteners.

DON'T GIVE UP, GOOD SLEEP WILL CONTROL
YOUR EMOTIONAL SYMPTOMS FOREVER.

Case History
Number One

The Story of Jenny

When Jenny came to me, she was a 16-year-old high school girl who had a history of childhood bedwetting until puberty and who had suffered from chronic fatigue and a variety of sleeping disorders even before puberty. After she began to menstruate, it grew increasingly difficult for her to get up in the mornings. Concerned, her mother would usually let her sleep in on the weekends, hoping this would provide the additional rest she seemed to need. Although she did fairly well in school, the teachers told her parents that Jenny was a very moody and irritable girl, that she was having trouble making friends, and that she would cry easily over the smallest trifles.

As she passed through the years of puberty, Jenny became increasingly more emotional and hyper-sensitive. A school counselor tried to console her by telling her this was normally a bad time for most teenagers, especially for girls going through the delicate transition of becoming women, a time when their hormones were in flux. Accordingly, the counselor told her parents not to worry, just to relax and keep the lines of communication open.

While it was, admittedly, all too easy to equate Jenny's erratic mood swings with the typical problems encountered by most adolescents, Jenny's mother soon noticed there was a cyclic pattern to Jenny's behavior. She would invariably be much more depressed and irritable just before her period. She was also having menstrual cramps, which appeared to be fairly common in this age group, though they were probably not related to PMS. Her mother also observed marked changes in Jenny's attitude towards her friends during this time of the month. She was testy and would quarrel easily, or she would weep unaccountably over movies that really weren't that sad.

In time, she stopped talking or sharing with her parents, refusing to confide in them as she had done in early childhood. When her mother read a magazine article about PMS, she was struck by how closely the symptoms described matched Jenny's. She felt sure her daughter was suffering from this disease, even though everything else she had read on the subject suggested it was mostly older women who were bothered with this problem. As it happened, Jenny also had a younger sister, Karen, aged 11, who was a bedwetter and was having similar problems of fatigue and sleep deprivation.

When the girls' mother came to me with her two daughters, I placed both girls on my Tryptophan Treatment Program. Within a very short time, the 11-year-old stopped wetting the bed and raised her energy level by improving the quality of her sleep. Then, after a six month treatment plan, Jenny's mood swings and cyclical depressions completely disappeared. She also got along better with her friends, began to socialize more easily and established a stronger relationship with her parents.

Once again, this convinced me that my plan of treatment works for women of all ages—those just starting out, as well as those trying to make it through to menopause in one piece.

5

Facts About Menstruation

The Joys of Being a Woman

WHEN I LOOK BACK on the problems I have had with my own menstrual cycle, most of them being in the premenstrual phase, I wonder why I was so enthused at the idea of "starting" at age 12. I'm sure modern technology has made the whole experience a little easier with the invention of pads and tampons, but all in all it has definitely not been one of my best life experiences!

In order to understand why women with PMS experience abnormal changes in their menstrual cycles it is first important to look at what is normal. In terms of menstruation "normal" refers to a range of conditions.

The Normal Menstrual Cycle

The menstrual cycle is determined by the interaction of hormones which originate in the hypothalmus, the pituitary and the ovary. Two of these hormones, estrogen and progesterone, cause the uterine endometrium to proliferate, become secretory and eventually slough. More simply, these hormones cause the uterus to first fill with blood, and then secrete it.

For our purposes in this book, let's agree that the average period for the normal menstrual cycle is about 28 days. But this can range from 21 to 35 days. The number 28 is the result of the statistical averaging in which the cycle lengths of thousands of women were added together, then divided by the number of women counted. If, for example, half the women polled had 15-day cycles, and the others had cycles of 41 days, the average would be 28, even though perhaps none of the women had a 28 day cycle. Of course, women do experience cycles which are 28 days long, but few have such cycles every month.

Early in the menstrual cycle the pituitary releases a chemical called follicle stimulating hormone, or FSH, which stimulates primordial follicles to begin to grow in the ovary. As these follicles grow under the influence of FSH and small amounts of luteinizing hormones, or LH, they begin to secrete estrogens. These estrogens cause the endometrium (the lining of the uterus) to begin to grow and thicken. This is known as the proliferative phase of the menstrual cycle.

The process here is as follows:

This is the stage where the endometrium, or the lining of the uterus, begins to build up the supply of blood during the first half of the cycle. In this half of the cycle, the uterus is preparing hopefully for an egg to implant into the wall to create pregnancy. The tissue that has built up in the uterus is to help feed that possible pregnancy.

The rising levels of estrogen also affect the production of pituitary gonadotropins. The increased levels of estrogen cause suppression of FSH, which, in turn, causes a rise in estrogen until, when it reaches a certain point, it starts to suppress the FSH, and thus is produced a negative feedback system.

At approximately day 14 of a 28-day cycle, the combined action of a surge of LH and a small amount of FSH, still being released by the pituitary, brings the ovarian follicle to maturity. The ripened follicle releases an ovum and ovulation has occurred.

Under the continuing influence of LH, the thin epithelial membrane is converted into a thick, folded, and firm glandular body, bright orange in color, and known as the corpus luteum. The luteal cells of this ovarian gland secrete a second hormone known as progesterone. This converts the proliferative endometrium into a secretory type which is well suited to receive a fertilized ovum. Should the ovum fail to become fertilized, the rising levels of ovarian hormones will exert a negative feedback effect on gonadotropin production by the pituitary, at which time the suppression of LH will occur. Deprived of hormonal support, the corpus luteum shrivels and dies. This in turn, leads to deterioration of the endometrium and, eventually, to menstruation.

The Causes for Cycle Fluctuations

For reasons that need have nothing to do with pregnancy, stressful episodes can either cause a women to be unusually late with her period or, in cases of severe shock, skip her cycle completely. For example, during the Holocaust many female prisoners of the concentration camps ceased to menstruate until they were liberated in 1945.

This wasn't due only to traumatic shock, however. These women had also been systematically starved, and thus a loss of body fat was involved. Estrogen is stored in body fat, and when the percentage of body fat becomes too low, as in the case of anorexic women, women stop menstruating. They are unable to produce the estrogen because they don't have enough fatty tissue.

It is interesting to note here that this phenomenon also occurs at present with some female athletes. Because of rigid training they actually train themselves into a state that is similar to menopause, insofar as they may develop a bone disease called osteoporosis due to inadequate levels of estrogen. During rigid training periods, their percentage of body fat is down so low, and their muscle mass is so high that they are unable to menstruate. In developing osteoporosis, they lose the density of their bones, until their bone mass can't support their muscle mass. As a result, it becomes a process that is really working against their goals of perfect fitness and health.

Is There A "Normal" Amount of Blood-Flow During Menstruation?

Because so much of the process of menstruation is hidden—physically, psychologically and culturally—any changes in bleeding patterns will usually provoke some kind of anxiety. To say that no two women bleed alike wouldn't be accurate either, since so little research has been done on the variation of bloodflow with regard to age or any environmental factors. However, we can say that menstrual flow is real blood, and differs from other blood in our bodies insofar as it does not clot.

The average amount of blood that leaves the uterus during menstruation is about two ounces in each cycle, while the normal range of blood loss is anywhere from one to six ounces. This flow should in no way be alarming, as it does not lead to anemia.

Under normal conditions, variations in bleeding patterns are quite ordinary. But with so much variability, it's difficult for one to decide when a bleeding irregularity is normal and when it is something to worry about. The normal range of flow is from three to seven days; so if you think an eight-day flow is a symptom of a more serious problem, the best advice I can give you is to see your physician for a necessary blood test and examination.

Early Ovulation in Women With PMS

In March of 1985, a study done by J.F. Watt and Associates was published in the *British Journal of Obstet-*

rics and Gynecology. In this study, tests were done on women with PMS and women who were free of symptoms of PMS. It was found that the PMS patients appeared to ovulate approximately three days sooner than the control groups (those women who did not suffer symptoms of PMS). The PMS women ovulated on day 11 instead of day 14 as did the women in the control group. However, the significant point here is that the luteal phase (the period of time from ovulation to day one of the menstrual cycle) was 17 days instead of the normal 14 days. Prior to this study, it was always thought that no matter how long the menstrual cycle, the luteal phase was always 14 days. This early ovulation is also significant because it causes subtle changes in the normal estrogen/progesterone levels. Please see chart for a more visual explanation.

Previous PMS theories suggested that progesterone levels were too low in relationship to estrogen levels. However, although their appears to be a change in these levels it is because of this lengthened luteal phase. I believe that progesterone levels are low in relationship to estrogen levels when measured at the end of the menstrual cycle. However, as you will see these levels are actually controlled a step higher in the system, that is, in the brain by serotonin.

The suggestion with this study is that PMS patients' progesterone levels are actually peaking at a different time than women with normal menstrual cycles. That is, these levels are being stretched out for an additional three days. Because serotonin acts as a block, actually inhibiting luteinizing hormone in the brain, if the serotonin is too low it will not be able to effectively inhibit LH. The LH will surge too early causing early ovulation

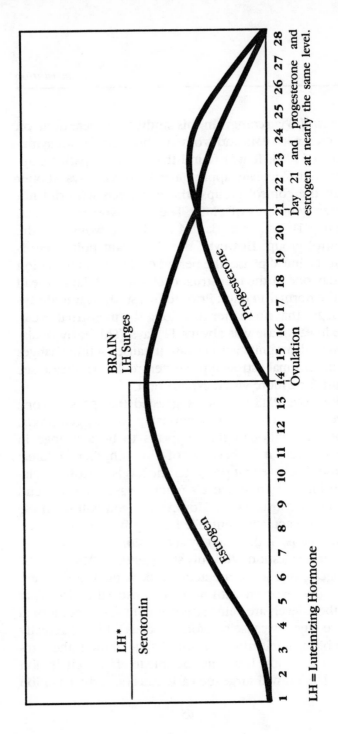

Normal Menstrual Cycle

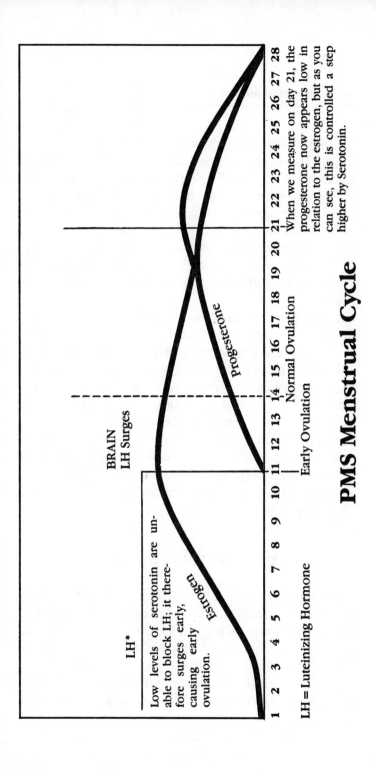

PMS Menstrual Cycle

LH*

Low levels of serotonin are unable to block LH; it therefore surges early, causing early ovulation.

LH = Luteinizing Hormone

BRAIN LH Surges

Estrogen

Progesterone

Early Ovulation

Normal Ovulation

When we measure on day 21, the progesterone now appears low in relation to the estrogen, but as you can see, this is controlled a step higher by Serotonin.

1 2 3 4 5 6 7 8 9 10 11 12 13 14 15 16 17 18 19 20 21 22 23 24 25 26 27 28

and subsequent changes in the estrogen/progesterone ratios. These changes in the estrogen/progesterone probably are responsible for the physical symptoms experienced by women with PMS. Such symptoms as breast tenderness, bloating, acne, etc. This study also showed that women with PMS tended to have smaller, immature ovum when compared to the control group of women, further supporting their theory that PMS women have early ovulation and an extended luteal phase.

If, however, the brain serotonin is increased over a period of time, a woman with PMS should then begin to ovulate at the correct time, when this happens physical symptoms are alleviated. It has been my experience with myself and other women I have treated for PMS that the physical symptoms seem to take a little longer to go away than do the emotional symptoms. However, within six months these symptoms should be entirely gone, assuming you are following the program as suggested. I no longer suffer any breast tenderness, bloating, acne or any other of the annoying physical PMS symptoms.

Previous PMS Theories

Premenstrual tension was first described in 1931 by R. T. Frank. Then, some 20 years later, in England, Dr. Katharina Dalton, while working with PMS patients, began to use the term "premenstrual syndrome" to cover this multitude of symptoms.

Dr. Frank wrote, "The group of women to whom I refer especially complained of a feeling of indescribable tension from ten to seven days preceding menstruation, which in most instances continues until the time that the menstrual flow occurs. The patients complain of unrest, irritability and the compulsive urge to find relief by a variety of foolish and ill-considered activities. Their personal suffering is intense and manifests itself in many reckless and sometimes reprehensible actions. Not only do they realize their own suffering, but they feel conscience-stricken towards their husbands and their families, knowing very well that they are being unbearable in both their attitude and behavior. Within an hour or two after the onset of the menstrual flow, complete relief from both physical and mental tension occurs."

My findings, however, are that the symptoms aren't always abated during the very beginning of menstruation. Under certain conditions, some women—myself included—will often have continuing symptoms following the start of their menstrual flow, perhaps lasting for another day or two.

It has been my experience that the mood swings are uppermost in importance, as these are the symptoms that do most to influence interpersonal relationships and the ability to cope with family members. They have the strongest bearing on the quality of our lives.

It's important for us to differentiate between those women who are truly suffering from PMS and those who may be suffering from a variety of other ailments, like thyroid problems or severe mental depression. The symptoms of so many emotional disturbances are so similar, I caution women to first make sure it's really PMS that's troubling them before they start on the Tryptophan Treatment Program. The best way to determine this is to chart these symptoms for a month or two.

To play it safe, before beginning this program I ask that women first see their own personal physician or practitioner.

The Causes of PMS

In the past there have been several theories as to what causes PMS. Each theory has generated its own solution(s) none of which has proven to be the definitive one, and all of which vary broadly in effectiveness.

Sex Steroids

Dr. Katharina Dalton developed the theory that PMS is caused by a hormonal imbalance in which there is too little progesterone in relation to estrogen. This imbalance can occur in two ways: an over-abundance of estrogen may be produced in the follicular (pre-ovulatory) phase of the cycle, swamping the system and blocking the functions of progesterone produced in the luteal phase. There is also the possibility that normal amounts of estrogen are produced during the follicular phase, but that less than average amounts of progesterone are manufactured in the luteal phase.

Dalton has written many books on PMS and has treated many women for the disease. She theorizes that when natural progesterone is used, the remission of symptoms is almost 100% assured. Synthetic progesterone has also been used as a treatment. However, it has proven to be ineffective in most cases. In Dr. Dalton's opinion, natural progesterone is the only positive treatment.

My own experience and recent studies indicate that there are problems with Dalton's theory. In my own case, progesterone was not the answer. Later I discovered that this treatment also had a "hit or miss" effect on many of my patients, and it seemed that no two patients taking the same dosage would have the same responses. Recent double blind studies using progesterone and a placebo, show no improvement with progesterone over the placebo. When I compare that sort of reaction to the very positive results of my Tryptophan Treatment Program, there's no question that the progesterone treatment theory has already become obsolete.

Although I would agree with Dalton that the progesterone is probably low in the later half of the luteal phase, I believe that the administration of progesterone is not the answer. As I previously pointed out this change in the estrogen/progesterone ratio is controlled a step higher in the system. With the correction of this brain chemical imbalance the progesterone will naturally normalize, and symptoms will disappear. I have also found that the Tryptophan Treatment Program should not be used in combination with progesterone as it is not as effective. For maximum results a woman should be on the program suggested in this book.

And yet, it must be noted that it was mostly Dalton's early findings that first focused any public attention on PMS. Because so few of the most esteemed gynecologists or endorinologists were taking PMS seriously at the time, however, Dalton was fighting a lonely battle.

Vitamin Therapy

There have been numerous studies linking the symptoms of PMS to vitamin deficiencies, especially vitamin B_6. Many researchers believe that vitamin B_6 is an important factor in the synthesis of both serotonin and dopamine. Some researchers suggested very large doses for treatment, however, in large doses Vitamin B_6 has been found to cause some nerve damage. Many women experienced some relief of symptoms with B_6, because B_6 is necessary to convert tryptophan to serotonin. However, it alone will not eliminate PMS symptoms.

There have been numerous PMS multi-vitamins on the market, among them Optivite and Dr. Susan Lark's formula. These vitamins are high in the B vitamins, calcium, magnesium and niacinamide as well as other vitamins. For many women they have offered a measure of relief. The reason, in my opinion, is primarily their relationship to serotonin and sleep. As I mentioned above, B_6 is necessary to make serotonin. By ingesting large amounts of niacinamide (or nicotinic acid) we fill up that pathway and allow the tryptophan that is present in our diet to be shunted to the serotonin pathway. See chart for visual clarification (pp. 41 and 42). Calcium and magnesium are both necessary for normal restful sleep.

I think it is clear to most women suffering from PMS

that, although vitamins are essential and may improve PMS, they do not completely eliminate the symptoms. The Tryptophan Treatment Program combines the necessary vitamins with the necessary amino acid to eliminate PMS symptoms completely.

Fluid Retention

One of the most prevalent theories several years ago was that fluid retention caused PMS. It was thought that irritability was a result of a slight increase in fluid on the brain which caused emotional symptoms. Many doctors have tried giving diuretics as a treatment for this fluid retention; although some improvement in bloating has been noticed, other symptoms have not improved. Diuretics can also be potentially harmful as many deplete stores of necessary potassium. I have found that diuretics are not necessary in the treatment of PMS. Those physical symptoms such as bloating and breast tenderness will disappear after a time on the Tryptophan Treatment Program.

Endorphins

At present a very popular hypothesis relates to endorphins. Endorphins are the brain's own morphine surrogate, so to speak. We create endorphins in the brain by certain kinds of strenuous physical involvement, like exercise. After there has been a certain amount of physical energy-output, usually taking you well past your normal limits, it is the endorphins working in the brain that cause you to feel that heightened sense of well being or euphoria. This is why some people exercise so devotedly, hoping to achieve that inimitable "high" they can only get from this endorphin kick. As a result, some people become addicted to this good feeling by running marathon races, riding exercise bikes, or performing aerobics.

But there is another side to this coin which is called endorphin withdrawal, and this has been suggested as another reason why some women are suffering more severe PMS symptoms in recent years. When a person has been experiencing a high level of endorphin output for a long period, and there is a sudden reversal causing this level to decline, the suggestion by researchers has been that PMS symptoms then occur. And yet, interestingly enough, lowered levels of endorphins are associated with low levels of serotonin. In fact, the endorphin level is probably lower during PMS, which is why some women claim to feel much better if they exercise strenuously during this time.

Prostaglandins

While prostaglandins might sound like the name of an obscure village in Outer Mongolia, it turns out to be another chemical that has been suggested as a cause for both PMS and menstrual cramps. Some researchers have suggested the use of a chemical called Evening Primrose which affects the levels of certain prostoglandins. Although I and many of my patients tried this approach the results were disappointing.

While increased levels of prostaglandins are also associated with menstrual cramps, it is interesting to note that there does not appear to be a correlation between those women who suffer from PMS and those who suffer with menstrual cramps. It appears a woman is more likely to have either one or the other, although some unfortunate souls suffer from both.

It is believed that the main cause of menstrual cramps is, in fact, higher levels of prostaglandins. These levels can be very easily controlled with anti-inflammatory/anti-prostaglandin medications, such as Motrin or Anaprox. These are prescription medications which when used correctly should control menstrual cramps. For good results they must be started a day or two before the menstrual period begins and continued for a few days into the period. I myself had very little experience with menstrual cramps; however, that was about the only unpleasant premenstrual symptom I did not have. Because tryptophan is so effective in pain control, it has also proven to be an important adjunct in the control of menstrual cramps. Many of my patients have had complete relief of menstrual cramps on this program alone.

Many of the theories that I have mentioned, as well as others which are less significant, are really in my opinion pieces of the greater PMS puzzle. Although, each theory addresses a few sypmtoms, the Premenstrual Solution is the only one that addresses them all.

Case History
Number Two

The Story of Noreen

Noreen is now 33 years old. She had a history of childhood bedwetting until the age of 11. When she first came to me, she had the following story to tell:

"Although I never knew what to call it until now, I guess PMS has virtually ruined my life. For many years I was certain I was on the verge of losing my mind, and so were a lot of other people. That's why I've been treated for mental illness off and on since I was about seventeen. I've taken every major tranquilizer, sedative and antidepressant on the market. Thorazine, librium, valium, and that's just for starters. I have been diagnosed by shrinks, neurologists, therapists, and they all agreed I was a paranoid schizophrenic with suicidal tendencies.

"Incredible as it sounds, it wasn't until about four years ago that any of those experts noticed the connection between my mental health hospitalizations and my menstrual cycle. And yet the first day of my hospital stay practically always coincided with the onset of my period. I can't even count how many times I ended up in some psycho ward for suicide attempts. I was getting very good at slashing my wrists, though maybe I was just trying to get the right attention from someone, knowing some member of my family would find me before I bled to death. I remember shouting outrageous obscenities at the paramedics whenever they dragged me out of the house.

"I was so full of rage, I hated everybody I saw. Even when I was able to remain at home, during the two weeks before my period, I was bedridden most of the time. I remember times when, while walking down the street, I would have these violent and destructive feelings, like I wanted to machine-gun everyone in sight. Or I would go into the most awful screaming fits in public, or in department stores, yelling the most filthy insults at some of the clerks, accusing them of ignoring me or not being polite enough . . ."

It came as no surprise to me when Noreen told me that she had never been married. Furthermore, due to her PMS symptoms, she had never been able to sustain any prolonged relationship with a man. When she first came to me she was—as she had been for most of her adult life—unemployed. Indeed, by that time she had become unemployable. She'd also had problems coping in high school, and finally had to drop out. Whenever an exam fell the week before her period, she would have to call in sick, and miss school for several days.

She told me that, in general, her premenstrual problems occured during the last two weeks before her period. But she added: "If I have any change in my sleep patterns, or if I'm unable to sleep for a few days, at any time of the month, I'll start getting 'flashback symptoms.' You know, like it's my period all over again, even at times when I know it isn't."

Naturally, this patient was far more concerned with her psychological symptoms than her physical symptoms. As she put it, "I guess this is what happens when a bunch of big-time medicine men treat you like a nut case for so many years. I mean, who was *I* to doubt the diagnoses of all those experts?"

Fortunately, there is a happy ending to this horror story. After being on my Tryptophan Treatment Program six weeks, Noreen was able to perform in a much more normal capacity. After three months on the program, she was improved enough to hold down a full-time job for the first time in her life. And now, after more than six months on the treatment, she happily reports that she considers herself to be about 95% improved.

Furthermore she is no longer taking tranquilizers, antidepressants or any any other form of prescription drugs.

6

Yesterday's Myths Versus Today's Realities

Most of Those Old Wives' Tales About PMS Were Started by Old Husbands

IN THE PAST, there have been countless weird and irrational taboos regarding menstruation. In one ancient society it was believed that if a man ever cast his eyes upon menstrual blood, he would immediately be struck blind. There were still other cultures where it was firmly believed that the menstruating female was a castrated and bleeding male in another incarnation, and that if any man came in contact with a menstruating woman, he would have to sacrifice his own male genitalia as punishment.

Other philosophers—all of them men, it must be noted—describe menstrual blood as a kind of all-purpose poison, even an effective insecticide, able to destroy various bugs, shrivel up the seeds of garden flowers, and even cause fruits to rot on their branches and drop from the trees in disgrace. And thus, the evolution of "the curse" began.

Among the ancient Persians, it was believed that "normal" menstruation should only last about four days. If a woman was still engaged in her "dirty business" at the end of that period, she was given a hundred lashes and sent back into isolation for five more days. If she was still menstruating at the end of this time, she was given 400 lashes because she was possessed by demonic spirits.

In general, the act of menstruation implied that a woman was being punished for some reason, possibly for some "unclean" deed she had performed in another life. For this reason she was taken away from the main house during her cycle and locked into a separate hut or some other remote place of solitary confinement safely removed from the more fastidious male members of the tribe. In addition, premenstrual problems might also explain why there were so many harems in ancient times. This enabled the sultan or the caliph to rotate his "flock" more conveniently, depending on which of his brides was premenstrually indisposed. Ironically, however, women who live together often begin to cycle together.

In our society, it's true we don't *consciously* categorize menstruation as an evil, unclean function. For instance, few modern men who prefer not to have sexual intercourse during menstruation will regard this as protection against either demonic forces or the threat of castration. It is more likely they will attribute this preference to respect for the woman. Some of today's most sophisticated and cosmopolitan males would especially laugh at the notion that they are still governed by some atavistic aversion to the process of menstruation or that they view it as something fearful, spooky or dangerous. On the contrary, some of the more enlightened ones would insist on proximity and even intimacy during this time. However, many men will still manage to politely keep their distance during the menstrual period, both before and during. This implies that even today, in the super-liberated eighties, old fears and superstitions remain. As such, they still need to be put down.

Lamentably, for women as well as men, these old taboos often have a lingering, residual effect. For some women—perhaps those who were never too hot for sexual equality in the first place—the old belief that menstruation is "dirty," or at the least, "not very nice" only serves to reinforce their own negative self images. And thus, it becomes all too easy to revive the instinctive shame they feel about their body's secretive and unmentionable processes, reminding them anew that they are the most "defective" of the two sexes. This might explain why so many of today's women help to keep the concept of PMS locked in the closet: when given the choice, such women will still prefer to seek the advice of a male rather than a female specialist. It's as if at the very simplest level they are saying, "How can I expect a mere woman to help me with this problem, when she's just as defective (unworthy) as I am?"

Naturally, I don't mean to suggest that menstruation is a glandular Shangri-la. But it *is* a fact of life, and a very human fact. What it is *not*, however, is any form of biblical and/or voodoo punishment inflicted upon all females for the sole crime of *not being male*.

Why PMS Is More Extreme in the Eighties

From all my past research, I have learned that menstruation is a perfectly healthy process. What I now believe, however, is that premenstrual distress may be more prevalent during the past 30 years than at any time in recorded history.

I'm fairly sure PMS was around long before Frank's definition of it in 1931, but I suspect that the age-old taboos against "reporting" these symptoms kept it under wraps. Nevertheless, due to the advent of modern stress and technology, it seems logical to hypothesize that PMS symptoms are much more severe and widespread now than they were back in Grandma's day.

We know, for example, that 40 or 50 years ago women gave birth with far more frequency than they do now, due to the lack of contraception as well as to the cultural definition of most females as wives and mothers. Since then there have been a number of drastic cultural changes including such precedent-shattering developments as "the pill," equal rights for women, legalized abortion, as well as the recent tendency for married women to put off having children sometimes until their mid or late thirties. And even when they do have children, few contemporary women will have nearly as many children as their ancestors did.

In comparison the average woman during the early part of this century gave birth as often as seven, eight or even more times during her lifetime. During that era, being pregnant was a way of life for most women during the childbearing years. Thus, it stands to reason that if they spent about 85% of those years either being pregnant, giving birth or nursing, which usually suppresses the menstrual cycle, they wouldn't have been bothered by the process of menstruation often enough to think of it as a problem.

If, in a period of ten years, a woman has three pregnancies and nurses each child for approximately two years, she may have only 12–20 menstrual cycles. But if, given the same time frame, the same woman has no pregnancies, she may have as many as 120 menstrual cycles. Therefore, in comparison to today's women, women of 50 or 60 years ago simply did not experience very many menstrual cycles by the time they were ready for menopause. As a result, except for those maiden ladies who may have suffered in silence for centuries, women then, because they didn't menstruate nearly as often as they do in the 80's, may not have suffered the special problems of PMS to the same extent as their modern counterparts.

When we draw these comparisons, we can only wonder if this could be the price we are paying for easier methods of birth control, the decision to have fewer children and to have them later and the legalization of abortion. More periods and fewer babies create the perfect environment for a greater incidence of PMS.

Don't get me wrong; I'm certainly not recommending pregnancy as a treatment for PMS. I am merely observing that PMS is *probably* more prevalent today than it was in the past and, therefore, must be reckoned with.

PMS and Women in the Work Force

To further support my theory that PMS is more prevalent in the 80's than it was in the past, let's remember that today's woman deals with more stress than ever before. She is often running two worlds concurrently if she handles an outside job and has a house and family to manage as well. In part, this is due to the vast changes in our economics in the past 15 years. With present-day inflation, there are few women who can afford to stay home, keep house and raise the kids. No longer is one salary enough for most households. And this, incidentally, adds more pressure for the working woman than the working husband. Studies show that even though the wife works, there is not necessarily a commensurate reapportioning of home responsibilities. She then has two jobs, while he only has one, which means there is double the amount of tension in her daily routine than in her husband's. If the monthly distress of severe PMS is added, pressures will mount exponentially.

Whether women want to work or must of necessity work, the result is always the same: more stress. Consequently, in this decade, it has been estimated that 70 to 90% of all women admit to having recurring PMS symptoms, while 20 to 40% suffer with such severity, it affects their jobs, their relationships and their ability to cope in society.

It has also been estimated that U.S. industry loses $30 billion annually, or 8% of their entire wage costs, because of disabilities associated with PMS. In view of these staggering statistics, it seems even more incredible that no serious studies were done on this problem years ago. I began to wonder if my proposed Tryptophan Treatment Program might not have more helpful repercussions than I ever anticipated. Not only will it be the solution for countless PMS sufferers, but also an industrial boon. With corrective treatment, there needn't be such vast numbers of women workers lessening their output or taking sick leave during certain times of the month.

PMS and Its Link to the Law: Are These Really Crimes of Passion?

In the past, much has been written about the increased incidence of mayhem and deviltry whenever there is a full moon. But that one night of lunar madness is but a drop in the bucket when compared to the number of crimes some women have committed during PMS. Although the statistics aren't nearly as abundant as those related to the cycle of the full moon, data collected over the years establishes a very real correlation between the crimes some women commit and the time of the month the are committed. Statistics stretching clear back to 1953 reveal that 62% of the inmates of a women's prison had committed their violent misdeed while in the throes of PMS. That was over 30 years ago, so one can well imagine how those figures must have escalated since then. In the United Kingdom, PMS is a justifiable murder defense, while in a few of our own states, it is now being accepted as a contributing factor in crimes of manslaughter, arson and assault. In France, PMS is officially recognized as a cause of temporary insanity and can often lead to a plea of diminished capacity and a suspended sentence in lieu of probation.

In this country, due to all the aforementioned taboos on this subject, the recurrences of criminal behavior related to PMS haven't exactly made front page headlines. But the law enforcement authorities we talked to came up with a consensus that went something like this:

"It's been my experience that most of the women in prison for killing their husbands or lovers have generally waited for that special time of the month to make their move. In fact, we locked up this one gal only a few weeks ago, and when one of the matrons asked her why she killed her old man, she said, 'The way I was feeling at the time, I wanted to kill everyone in sight. He just happened to be the only one handy.' As for this PMS you're talking about, now I wouldn't be surprised if that's what lit a fire under old Ma Barker fifty years ago, not to mention Lizzie Borden and her famous ax. But listen, if you think these ladies go ape once a month when they're on the outside, you should see what their periods do to them when they're locked up."

When we asked about the treatment these women received inside, we were told that in most cases they were heavily sedated or tranquilized, then left to sleep it off, sometimes in solitary confinement.

PMS victims don't live in a vacuum, so the scenario for domestic crime is potentially complex. For example, a PMS patient may be married to an alcoholic whose only method of dealing with her at "that time of the month" is to get "justifiably" drunk and beat her up. He can blame her for driving him to drink. Variations on this theme include rampant child abuse, the battered woman syndrome, incest, drug addiction, juvenile delinquency, joblessness and poverty, all of which could quite conceivably be happening in the household where the mother is suffering from severe

PMS symptoms. So there can be an endless combination of social problems in one household, all of them contributing to that final eruption that sends someone in the family to prison. Law enforcement agencies are powerless to control the chain reaction of PMS-related crimes until *after* the fact.

I would be willing to wager that (if potential female criminals had access to a PMS Treatment that really *treats* the disease instead of masking it), the population in our women's prisons would begin to drop off immeasurably.

Case History
Number Three

The Story of Elizabeth

Elizabeth is a 38-year-old female who is now married to her second husband. She believes that her previous divorce was a direct result of her severe PMS symptoms.

"But I didn't know that's what it was at the time," she told us. "It didn't start happening until about 10 years ago, after I had a late miscarriage. It was during the period right after my earlier divorce that I started having these screaming fits and temper tantrums. I have two children by my first husband, and when I caught myself physically abusing my youngest, I was so revolted and frightened, I started going to a psycho-therapist. I didn't tell him that I had attacked my own child, only that I had these frightening feelings of violence and that I felt I needed help to control them. At the time, I didn't think to tell the therapist what time of the month I had these feelings, nor even that they were cyclical. I was afraid if I mentioned anything about my menstruation, he might tell me what this other doctor told me the last time I went to someone for help. As soon as I mentioned having a difficult time during my period, he said, 'Oh, that's all it is, is it? Well then, that's my cue to give you the advice I give to all my ladies who are having this type of discomfort: "Go home, relax, and keep telling yourself, 'This, too, shall pass.' " '

"In time, I managed to stop being physically abusive to my youngest daughter, but during my PMS, I continued to inflict so much mental cruelty on both girls, I just know they will never understand or forgive me. I'm also afraid my youngest might tell her father about the times when I beat her, and then I would be involved in a custody battle; that's if he didn't prefer child-abuse charges against me, which he is fully capable of doing. Not that I blame him. I made him very unhappy, and was beginning to undermine my second marriage with similar behavior. I would get so paranoid premenstrually that I'd accuse my husband of cheating on me, telling him I was positive he didn't love me and that he never had. I would yell and curse at him, telling him how much I hated him, all the while listening to myself as if I were listening to some demented stranger. None of the things I yelled at him were true. He was the sweetest, most patient man, and I knew if I lost him because of this craziness, I wouldn't want to live. If that happened, I would let the girls' father have custody of them, and then I would take my own life."

Despite these symptoms, Elizabeth managed to work full time as a secretary. She said that during her good times, she would exhaust herself trying to make amends to her children for having been so vicious and abusive to them earlier. She added, "I got so tired of using the same old phrase, 'You know Mommy doesn't mean it when she's like that.' How long could I expect them to go along with that lame excuse?"

She spoke of one incident with her 13-year-old daughter when she had cooked a new casserole for dinner. At the time Elizabeth was on day 25 and was very irritable and tired, but she was determined to try this new casserole recipe. When she served the dinner, everybody seemed to enjoy the meal except her eldest daughter. She didn't care for it, and frankly admitted this to her mother. That put Elizabeth in an insane rage. She picked up the girl's plate of food and dumped it on her head, then screamed uncontrollably at her. She then ran out of the room into her bedroom where she flung herself on the bed and sobbed for more than an hour.

Obviously, this sort of behavior can have a serious effect on a child and throws the whole family into turmoil. Fortunately, Elizabeth came to me in time to save her marriage, her sanity, and her relationship with her children. After being on my treatment program approximately two months, she reported she was feeling improvement in her symptoms. After six months she noticed great improvements in both her symptoms and in her family's attitude towards her. Now, whenever she gets reasonably upset about something, they are no longer so quick to attribute it to her former PMS hangups.

7

HOW PMS Relates to Depression and Nutrition

Do Those Cravings Get You Down?

PMS and Depression

As I POINTED OUT EARLIER, depression is one of the most devastating symptoms of PMS. This depression can change a woman's entire perception of her life and her surroundings. It isn't really surprising to note that statistically, more women suffer from depression than do their male counterparts. The reason for this may, in fact be two-fold. First, women have lower levels of serotonin at least during the second half of their menstrual cycles. This lower level of serotonin is probably the primary factor in the statistic mentioned above.

Additionally, women are generally more apt to admit they are occasionally depressed, and this may color these statistics. Whether women suffer more depression than do men is probably not as important as the fact that millions of women all over the world are suffering to one degree or another.

I feel it is important to point out the wide range in severity of depression experienced by women suffering with PMS. Symptoms of depression vary greatly not only in intensity, but also in duration. For some women depression can be truly debilitating, lasting 17 or 18 days each month, actually inhibiting them from performing normal routine tasks. On the other hand, some women experience only a day or two of mild depression. Women often describe this as a dark cloud which appears and changes their perspective on every day events. For some women the risk of suicide is very real, while for other women their depression manifests itself as a mild annoyance. Regardless of the severity of the symptoms experienced by women with PMS, this problem need no longer be an issue.

In addition, there are many forms of depression besides those related to PMS depression. This, clearly, makes the diagnosis of depression versus PMS difficult. Many women who, in fact, are suffering from PMS have probably been misdiagnosed as chronically depressed. For example, if their symptoms last as long as 17 or 18 days each month followed by the menstrual period, they may have only seven to ten days when they are symptom-free. This may not be enough time for either their doctor or these women to realize the cyclic nature of their depression. To further confuse the diagnosis, some women are reluctant to discuss the cyclic nature of their symptoms with their doctor. In fact, some women refer to PMS only in the most euphemistic of terms: "You know Doctor, I've been feeling a little nervous and edgy lately." Perhaps, embarrassed to discuss anything "female" in the presence of her doctor, one woman recently blamed her monthly "skitishness" on nuclear fallout.

The importance of finding a practitioner with whom a woman can communicate, in an environment which she percieves as safe is, in my opinion, critical to every woman's health. It is imperative that a woman find a practitioner she can trust. If the problem is not correctly identified, the treatment can not be accurately prescribed. If a woman does not find her practitioner supportive in her quest for good, informed health care, then I would encourage her to seek a practitioner who is. There are many fine, understanding doctors and medical practitioners who *will* listen and assess a womans health care needs.

For our purposes, it is important to determine the kinds of depression which may be confused with PMS. Some depressions are biological or genetic. These depressions are biochemical in nature, rather than behavioral. This means that long term therapy is not as effective as medications, such as antidepressants. These patients are depressed for no discernible reason. The depth of their melancholia appears to have no connection to life events, and this depression is not cyclic in nature but present at all times. There have been no real life changing events to institute this depression such as the loss of a loved one or a change in their living environment. These people are feeling the results of changes in brain chemistry. And since this depression is a disease of brain chemistry, it stands to reason that drugs, such as antidepressants which work by altering brain chemicals (serotonin, as well as other brain chemicals), can offer the control these people need. Such people have biological depression in much the same way as certain people suffer from biological diabetes.

However, if the depression is "situational," as a result of a recent shock or emotional crisis, then this depression is not biochemical and can be treated quite effectively with counseling or psychotherapy. Many women suffering from the depression experienced with PMS may have a combination of a brain chemical problem and a situational depression. When the brain chemical problem is corrected, much of the depression will lift; however, if situational problems, such as a problem marriage or a history of child abuse, etc., still exist, they may need to be worked out with a qualified therapist. On the other hand, women who are suffering depression, only as a result of PMS, should find complete relief from their symptoms through the program as outlined in this book.

Many of the antidepressants affect levels of serotonin or other chemicals in the brain such as dopamine or norepinepherine by either increasing or decreasing them. It has been my experience that antidepressants or MAO inhibitors are not as effective in the treatment of PMS as is tryptophan, and they have undesirable side effects. The safest and most effective way to increase neuroserotonin is the oral administration of tryptophan. This increase in brain serotonin coupled with increased sleep is extremely effective in the elimination of biochemical depression associated with PMS.

PMS and Nutrition

Over the past several centuries there have been dramatic changes in our eating habits which may have influenced the present high incidence of PMS. Originally man was primarily a hunter and a gatherer. His diet consisted of game, fish, fowl and just about anything else he could catch; he also ate wild grains, roots, fruits, fungus and berries. These foods were eaten on an availability basis. That is, if they were available, they may have been eaten or stored for later consumption. Even so, he often ate one food at a time, as opposed to eating combinations of foods whose chemical makeups may have been altered through preservatives and processing. The first major change in man's food supply came about with the development of agriculture around 10,000 B.C. While the domestication of plants and animals enabled man to settle down and brought about some wonderful cultural advances, it didn't dramatically alter his diet except to make it more secure.

From generation to generation, the human body has proven itself to be remarkably flexible and adaptable, always managing to make the best of whatever food supply happened to be available. Perhaps the human machine has back up systems to handle just about any emergency except that of being bombarded by a constant surplus of food. Today's dieters tend to become very frustrated as they find out that the body has a way of protecting against what its instincts warn may be the beginning of a famine. The body's metabolism automatically slows to conserve "valuable" stored fat. It would seem that this is a survival instinct which was necessary for our ancestors who had to depend on hunting and gathering for their food supply, but has become nearly obsolete in today's society, at least for most Americans.

The American diet, in my opinion, is generally too high in fat (animal fat, in particular), sugar and sodium. It is probably too low in fresh vegetables, fruit, complex carbohydrates and fiber. Statistics show that the fat content in the average American diet is a whopping 40% of the calories consumed, and that the average American consumes 125 pounds of sugar every year. Much of this sugar, sodium and fat is hidden in processed foods. For our bodies, this kind of a diet results in a silent energy crisis. When combined with PMS, the consequences of a poor diet become even more critical.

I know that when my PMS was severe, food was the solace I often turned to. I found that my cravings for sugar and chocolate, as well as other carbohydrates, were so severe that it did not matter to me at all that I was consuming too large a quantity of sugar; I simply had to have it. Why? Because the craving for carbohydrates or protein is directly related to levels of serotonin in the brain. Serotonin actually controls whether we crave carbohydrates or protein. If the levels of neuroserotonin are too low, the brain tells the body to eat carbohydrates to raise these levels. As I mentioned earlier in this text, tryptophan is necessary in order to make serotonin. It would then seem logical that if we wanted to increase the amount of brain serotonin then it would be necessary to consume more protein, which contains tryptophan and the other amino acids. However, this is not true. (For more visual clarification, please refer to the adjoining charts.)

Here is how the brain controls our dietary cravings:

When a person ingests a protein which contains all of the essential amino acids, including tryptophan, these amino acids then move from the stomach into the intestines and are absorbed into the blood stream. These amino acids now have to compete with each other to cross what is known as the blood brain barrier. In order to cross the blood brain barrier, the amino acids must attach themselves to what is known as a carrier molecule, a molecule, which will help them slide easily into the brain. The problem here, however, is that the competition can be fierce! All the amino acids, including tryptophan, are trying to push each other to get in through the blood brain barrier.

Researchers at MIT found that when individuals were given a meal high in carbohydrates, which caused a surge of insulin in the body, all of the amino acids, with the exception of tryptophan, became literally paralyzed. Tryptophan has the unique ability to attach itself to a carrier molecule that insulates it from insulin, and it is the only amino acid that can accomplish this.

As a result, although there are no greater levels of tryptophan in the bloodstream, more becomes available to slide through to the brain simply because the competition has been effectively eliminated. Thus, when you eat a carbohydrate, whether it be simple such as candy, or complex such as a whole grain, the amount of tryptophan that crosses to the brain is increased. Because simple carbohydrates tend to raise insulin levels more quickly, it is my belief that women with PMS have been trying, in effect, to unconsciously

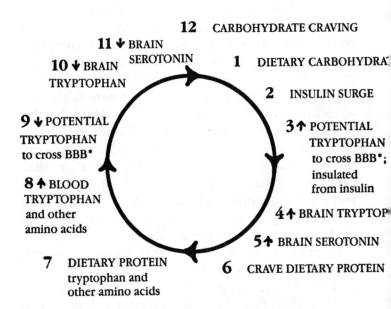

*Blood Brain Barrier

"Dietary Patterns"

1. Carbohydrate consumed.

2. Insulin surge secondary to carbohydrate consumption.

3. Tryptophan attaches itself to a protein molecule which insulates it from insulin. Other amino acids are unable to cross the blood-brain barrier in the presence of insulin. The competition for slots to cross the blood-brain barrier is decreased and more tryptophan crosses.

4. Increased levels of brain tryptophan occur.

5. Increased tryptophan allows an increase in the brain serotonin.

6. Increased levels of brain serotonin cause cravings for dietary protein.

7. Dietary protein is consumed.

8. There is an increase in blood tryptophan and other amino acids.

9. Increased competition with other amino acids makes it more difficult for tryptophan to cross the blood-brain barrier.

10. Decreased brain tryptophan.

11. Decreased brain serotonin.

12. Carbohydrate craving, then consumption of dietary carbohydrate.

Brain

Diagram 1

Blood Brain Barrier

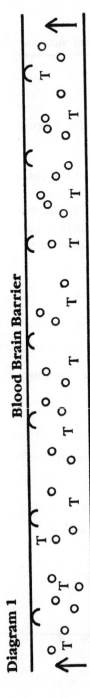

o = other amino acids trying to compete to cross the blood brain barrier and enter the brain

T = Tryptophan also trying to compete to enter the brain through the blood brain barrier

Brain

Diagram 2

Blood Brain Barrier

• = other amino acids which have now become paralyzed in the presence of insulin and unable to compete to cross into the brain

T = Tryptophan; although there is no more tryptophan in the blood, because there is less competition, tryptophan can now cross easily. This will in turn make more tryptophan available and will increase brain serotonin.

raise their levels of brain serotonin. It was my experience that eating sugar did in fact help my symptoms, but the improvement was very brief and transient. My body would then have to cope with the problem of my blood sugar bouncing up and down. PMS researchers have long thought that changes in blood sugar were associated with symptoms. I believe that the changes stem from chronically low levels of brain serotonin in women with PMS. Women are unable to effectively raise these levels of serotonin high enough to cause a craving for protein. The Tryptophan Treatment Program creates a way to effectively increase the brain tryptophan and thus increase the brain serotonin which will normalize this dietary pattern and thus neutralize this craving forever.

A complete lack of tryptophan in the diet can cause a disease called pellagra. This disease in prominent only in underdeveloped countries, whose main dietary staple is corn. The interesting point here is that the emotional symptoms are nearly identical to those experienced by women with PMS, and by people suffering from sleep deprivation. Diets which are based primarily on corn are lacking in either tryptophan or niacin (Tryptophan is necessary in order to make niacin or nicotinic acid, see Chart pp. 41 and 42). Denied this essential amino acid, these natives develop pellagra.

The symptoms of pellagra are general nervousness, mental confusion, depression, apathy, rage, delirium and severe sleep-deprivation. I find it interesting to note that when an entire culture is deprived of this amino acid through dietary deprivation, women, more than men, particularly between the ages of 20 and 45 become symptomatic. This would indicate that menstruating women tend to have greater needs for tryptophan and are more susceptible to dietary deprivation of this amino acid. When patients with pellagra are placed on either tryptophan or niacin all emotional symptoms disappear within four or five days. This is the same amount of time it takes to recover from complete sleep deprivation.

It has become clear that our diets and food habits are strongly linked to whatever emotional crisis we may be facing at any given time. It is, therefore, necessary to make sensible food choices in order to help eliminate and control the symptoms of PMS.

The importance of moderation in our dietary planning is critical. Learning to combine good nutrition, moderation and satisfying food can offer a challenge, but the rewards of learning new ways to eat will benefit not only a woman's PMS but her general health and well being. A sound program of good nutrition should include complex carbohydrates. Somewhere between 60–70% of the daily calories should come from this source. Unfortunately, the American diet appears to be sorely lacking in complex carbohydrates and too high in simple carbohydrates such as sugar, etc. Complex carbohydrates are plentiful in all vegetables, fruits and whole grains such as rolled oats, brown rice, wheat, and unsweetened cereals. They are also found in legumes, seeds and nuts, as well as potatoes, and breads. I would highly recommend that these foods be increased to a minimum of 60% of the caloric content of a woman's diet. Proteins should make up approximately 15–20% of the total caloric content of a woman's food budget. The essential amino acids are found in complete proteins such as beef, fish, poultry, eggs, milk, yogurt and cheese. The body actually requires approximately 35–55 grams of protein per day, or between one and two ounces. By increasing complex carbohydrates and decreasing protein, we can facilitate an increase in brain serotonin as well as help prevent such diseases as heart disease, hypertension and diabetes. It is also extremely critical to watch the amount of fat consumed, as these calories can not only be detrimental to health, but also make up a great percentage of the caloric content in most American diets. The average American diet is composed of more that 40% fat and most of this is from animal fat, which is of greater concern because of the cholesterol content. Whenever possible, fat in the diet should be unsaturated, which means it does not contain cholesterol. The total percentage of fat in the diet should be not higher than 25% and slightly lower, if possible.

Since it is often difficult to begin to make dietary changes, it is best to start gradually and build up. Begin by adding additional complex carbohydrates to your diet, and reducing protein and fat slightly. Look at the positive effects these changes can make in your life and well being and that of your family. Change takes time and patience. Try new foods; experiment a little. Instead of viewing these dietary changes as a burden, look on them as a life-long commitment to better health. TAKE CARE OF YOUR BODY, AND YOUR BODY WILL BEGIN TO TAKE CARE OF YOU.

GOOD NUTRITION IS ESSENTIAL for good health and the elimination of PMS. Here are some helpful nutrition do's and don't's.

NUTRITION DO's

Do eat regular meals.
Do eat whole grains, pasta, potatoes, brown rice and breads.
Do eat fresh vegetables and fruits.
Do eat fish and chicken.
Do eat minimal amounts of animal protein.
Do avoid fat, particularly unsaturated fats.
Do avoid sodium (salt).
Do consider food as fuel for your body.
Do try new foods.
Do eat a wide variety of foods.
Do eat with family and friends whenever possible.
Do chew your food well.
Do enjoy your food and concentrate on what you are eating.
Do eat foods you enjoy, providing they are healthy.
Do eat when you are hungry.
Do eat slowly.
Do use moderation in your consumption of alcohol and caffeine.

NUTRITION DON'T's

DON'T USE ARTIFICIAL SWEETENERS.
Don't eat fast foods.

Don't go on fad diets, instead exercise good nutritional judgment.

Don't use food as a source of comfort.

Don't overeat.

Don't eat when you are full.

Don't expect to change your diet overnight, change takes time.

Don't clean your plate. If you have had enough, stop eating.

Don't eat while you watch TV or read.

Don't attempt a weight loss program until your PMS is in control.

Don't eat large quantities of simple carbohydrates.

Don't forget your multivitamins and multiminerals.

Don't be afraid to try new foods.

Case History
Number Four

The Story of Denise

Denise is a 44-year-old female who had been suffering from severe PMS for 15 years when she came to me for treatment. She'd had three pregnancies in the past, followed by a tubal ligation to prevent future pregnancies. After this procedure, she noticed a marked increase in her symptoms. Over the years, she sought the advice and treatment of several gynecologists, experimenting with progesterone, diuretics, vitamin therapy, hypnosis, acupuncture and even chiropractic care. But she had never gotten anything but the most minimal relief from any of her symptoms.

At present, now that she's able to laugh at her past miseries, she says, "I was so desperate, there was a time when I would have gladly tried a lobotomy, if I thought it would have helped. And I'm sure if I did, my husband and kids would have been cheering from the sidelines after they wheeled me out of the operating room, yelling, 'Way to go, Mom. Now that you're a vegetable, maybe we'll get more peace and quiet in our house!' "

She finally went to a specialist who convinced her that a hysterectomy was her only answer to this problem. But when she agreed to have a partial hysterectomy, which left her ovaries intact, she noticed very quickly that her PMS symptoms continued as before. Because she had pinned all her hopes on this surgery, its failure to alleviate her symptoms only added to her monthly distress. She also felt she had been deceived into thinking this would be her solution when, in fact, it only intensified the problem.

Because her husband and children showed no patience or understanding for her problem, the pressures mounted for her. Her husband belittled the whole situation and summed it up by saying, "I've just got one of those wives who's a pain in the ass once a month." Her children and other family members accused her of deliberately dramatizing her symptoms to attract sympathy and attention. Although Denise worked part-time and also did volunteer work, she found it more and more of an ordeal to cope.

She tried going on a program of estrogen supplementation which gave her some relief, though it didn't last very long. She would become increasingly more withdrawn from her friends each month, at which times she would invariably feel depressed and almost suicidal and would contrive loud and abusive arguments with her family over trifles. This behavior was so totally unlike her natural self, she began having very real fears for her sanity.

When Denise finally heard about my new treatment program, I knew after the first consultation that she had found me just in time, as she was truly desperate. Like the majority of my other patients, after Denise started on my program, she began improving steadily. At present, she is unable to tell exactly where she is in her cycle, for she no longer suffers all the old warning symptoms. She sleeps much better and awakens feeling rested and refreshed, and she adds: "I think my family is even happier than I am that I no longer have any of the aggravating symptoms I used to nag about in the past."

8

The Many Faces of Stress

Living a Life Free of PMS

THERE IS good stress and there is bad stress, and our bodies respond to both. The spirit of competition experienced by the athlete as he prepares for some challenging sporting event culminates in a primarily healthy form of stress. In practice, the athlete imposes stress on his body because he knows it will slowly respond by increasing its capacity. Thus, the boxer runs miles to increase his endurance, the football player lifts weights to increase his lean body mass, and the cross-country runner actually runs longer than required of him in the upcoming event to increase his over-all performance. The athlete uses self-imposed stress to his own advantage. He is in control. Bad stress produces the opposite effect by triggering effects over which the individual has no control. Stress caused by diet or the environment falls into the latter category and creates victims instead of victors.

Sometimes the relationship between good and bad stress can be subtle. The highly conditioned athlete who has purposefully subjected his body to physical stress may jeopardize the effects of all his physical training should he fail to take into account the mental training required to deal with the emotional demands of competition.

Fight or Flight

Early man was endowed with an elaborate system to deal with stress, a primal instinct which we think of as the fight or flight urge for survival. For example, if while stalking through the forest he was confronted by some dangerous predator like a sabre-toothed tiger, his emotional system would grow alert and wary, and he would prepare himself either to fight the foe or turn around and flee. During this process his entire metabolic rate would shoot up. His pulse rate would quicken, his adrenal glands would secrete adrenalin, his peripheral blood capillaries would constrict, elevating his blood pressure and blood flow to the brain. Other glands would secrete other hormones, his muscles mobilizing glycogen for quick energy needs, while other tissues mobilized fatty acids for long-term energy needs.

In many ways, this same sequence of events still prevails today.

Physical Stress

Physical stress takes on many forms other than that of the athlete applying stress to develop his body to its maximum potential. There are other forms of unexpected stress for which we cannot be prepared, like the trauma of a sudden traffic injury, or the stress faced by the non-athlete who finds he must run from a mugger or just to catch a train. Every year you hear of people dying from a sudden heart attack while shoveling snow, simply because their bodies were not equal to such rigorous tasks.

Physical stress places demands on our body for which we must be prepared. It stands to reason that the conditioned body can handle a sudden injury or a threatening encounter with a mugger more effectively than can the non-conditioned or "soft" body. In each case the body produces adrenalin, but if the heart is not equal to the task, you can forget about the "fight or flight" option, because then you're in no condition to do either.

We should all take a tip from the trained athlete who knows that all physical stress requires a planned program of conditioning.

Emotional Stress

To some extent, all stress is emotional. For example, in one study a physician gave a talk to a group of nurses. In this situation, since the nurses were his subordinates, he was in complete control. His pulse rate, blood pressure and metabolic rate remained constant. In short, he was relaxed and perfectly composed, not in the least rattled or on edge.

But when the doctor gave the same talk to a group of other physicians, his peers, some of whom had more seniority than he, he wasn't nearly so cool or controlled. In this set of circumstances his competency was on the line. Thus, the same speech produced quite different results. The doctor's pulse quickened, his blood pressure increased and his metabolic rate became elevated. He was, in short, under stress.

This is a perfect example of how emotional factors can have a physical effect on our bodies. Moreover, had the physician actually been in fear of losing his job, he might have perspired, or his throat might have gone suddenly very dry, or even the timbre of his voice might have altered.

There are other forms of emotional stress which can have overwhelming consequences, for example, the sudden death of a loved one, a divorce, the loss of a job, being rejected by a friend, the failure to pass an exam after much study, learning of an incurable illness, etc. Any of these events can place incredible emotional pressures upon the body, and in some cases, have caused serious, if not fatal, illness.

Equally as debilitating can be the daily on-the-job stress that plagues many people: deadlines, executive meetings, competition, job insecurity, etc. This is chronic stress that "comes with the territory." Indeed, many high-level executives, both male and female, appear to thrive on this type of stress and manifest no unhealthy symptoms. However, this kind of stress can be particularly intense for ambitious, upwardly mobile women with PMS, who, if their condition were known might be judged as potentially unreliable in a crisis. Women with PMS justifiably fear being branded as emotionally unstable by their bosses. They usually operate on the theory that public knowledge of their condition will jeopardize their careers. As a result, they are afraid to admit to having problems with PMS even with female coworkers.

Environmental Stress

In a previous chapter, we referred to the lady who attributed her PMS symptoms to nuclear fallout. Although she may have been stretching the point a bit, on one level she wasn't all that inaccurate. There are many forms of external stress over which we have little control. These are the pressures imposed upon us by our environment. For example, not many people realize that such things as air pollution or acid rain are forms of *toxic stress* as well as a possible source of toxic poisoning. In other words, before the proliferation of toxic waste dumps and other environmental threats succeed in killing us, they will first make us *very nervous.*

The same holds true for the oxidants emanating from heavy factory smoke, industrial fumes, the traffic residue we inhale while stuck in a freeway jam, the exhalations of a chain smoker with whom we might be trapped in an elevator.

All of these and many other environmental influences add up to stress as they take their toll on our bodies, physically and mentally. The physical stress is generated by the pollutants in the air, while the emotional stress results in our frustration and inability to deal effectively with those forces. Because we can neither change nor improve the situation, we feel trapped and futile.

Stress and Men's PMS Symptoms

I have recently discovered that PMS is not a problem for women only. The major symptoms of PMS originate from the brain, standard equipment for both men and women. This means that *we are all in this together*.

When I speak of men having PMS symptoms, I am not referring only to those caring husband who might be experiencing sympathy pains for their wives. The men I refer to needn't be married at all. Some men I have spoken to recently, a few of whom I have treated for this disease, are willing to admit to a list of symptoms very similar to those women with PMS complain about, symptoms which occur, if not cyclically, at least intermittently. I am not referring to "bio-rhythms" here, nor to mid-life crisis nor even to the full moon syndrome. Many of the men who experience PMS symptoms are in their twenties and thirties, and represent just about every walk of life.

As we have already observed, more men than women have a history of childhood bedwetting—60% as compared to 40% for women. And since bedwetting is a sleep disorder which creates emotional repercussions, it follows that more men than women were emotionally disturbed as children, and, thus, will be more susceptible to residual dysfunctions when they become adults.

However, while some men might suffer even more bad days of the month than their wives or lovers, few of them can or are willing to make the connection between their symptoms and a traditionally female condition. Because their symptoms are mainly psychological, and their bad days are not accompanied by the kind of somatic complaints which require an emergency run to the corner drug store, this can be a less noticeable malady for men than it is for women. Nevertheless, some men may suffer PMS symptoms as frequently as four out of every seven days.

The stressful symptoms we speak of are severe depression, erratic mood swings, unaccountable rages and temper tantrums, recurring tension headaches, inappropriate over reaction to trifling situations and, most defeating of all, chronic insomnia. Because these periodic symptoms are never connected to a man's sexual or hormonal functions—except for those men for whom the nervous fatigue created by insomnia seems to heighten their sex drive—there isn't the kind of stigma attached to a man's bad days as there is to a premenstrual woman's.

On the contrary, many men interpret their symptoms within a traditional male context. In which case the breadwinner might say when he gets home, "Now, don't mess with me tonight, kids. Daddy's under a lot of stress on the job. Lots of people depend on me, and I've got a lot of big decisions to make every day. So you guys just give me my space tonight, okay?"

This type of reaction reinforces the old double standard—when Daddy is tense or moody or short-tempered, he is to be admired, respected and comforted for carrying on in the line of duty. But when Mommy displays the same symptoms, she is considered a nag, a shrew, unreasonable and/or deficient.

The same double standard is mirrored in the marketplace. When a man is fiercely ambitious and stops at nothing to achieve success, he is often tremendously admired by his peers, and characterized as a "go-getter," "a tiger!" But when a business woman displays an equal amount of ambition, she runs the risk of being viewed as aggressive, unattractive, or compulsive.

Because stress is stress, no matter who feels it, many men who operate within long-term, successful, stressful situations will experience a decreased level of neuroserotonin, which decreases the quality of sleep, which in turn produces the emotional symptoms of PMS. This explains why my Tryptophan Treatment Program is now having the same excellent results with my male patients as it has had with my female patients.

In many cases, periods of stress can be far more intense for men than for women, especially those high-echelon executive types who carry the weight of the whole empire on their shoulders. These are the men who will also feel the need to suppress their softer feelings, and, thus, keep up a stoic and impenetrable front on the job. Usually, such suppression only heightens the tensions. And if these men are also working long hours, the result is constant fatigue, an overflow of adrenalin, which uses up the serotonin and causes changes in their sleep pattern. A combination of these factors makes it easy for a relatively minor frustration or crisis to trigger an overreaction on the job or at home.

How to Fight Stress with Exercise

On the subject of exercise, Robert Benchley once wrote, "Whenever I feel like exercising, I lie down until the feeling goes away."

Despite hordes of joggers sprinting in city parks, along streets and in the countryside, too many Americans still share Benchley's sentiments. Millions of sedentary types park their sports shoes on the coffee table while they watch T.V. They don't hear their arteries hardening nor do they think about the ramifications.

Nevertheless, the fact remains that some form of daily exercise is still one of the best ways to relieve stress or nervous tension. It also helps to prevent some of the degenerative cardiovascular diseases and high blood pressure. For women suffering with PMS, however, I recommend a more specialized regimen of exercise than for the general public.

Many forms of daily exercise will prove effective in combating your stress and relieving your PMS symptoms. However, the time of day you choose to exercise is very important. Because the Tryptophan Treatment Program is designed to increase the quality and quantity of a patient's sleep, I recommend as a first choice afternoon exercise, as this increases REM sleep. If you are unable to exercise in the afternoon because of your schedule then morning exercise is a good second choice as it has no effect on REM sleep. Evening exercise, particularly two hours prior to bedtime, decreases REM sleep and potentially will increase your PMS symptoms.

Initially, you might try a mild form of exercise such as walking, swimming or biking for a 20-minute period about three times a week. Although I feel certain that exercise is an important part of good health, I know from personal experience that women suffering with PMS have difficulty committing themselves to an exercise program. When my symptoms were very severe, I was too exhausted to even consider getting off the couch, much less trek to the gym. I personally had to feel better before I could start an intense exercise program. So don't get discouraged. Start slowly, and as you feel better, increase your physical activity.

For the PMS patient, regular exercise according to the time schedule suggested above will result in sounder and more refreshing sleep. In time, like everything else, a regular exercise program will become habit-forming. At the beginning it is important to start slowly exercising joints and muscles that perhaps haven't been used for years. A good policy is one small step at a time, rather than a fast quantum leap that could put you in traction before you've had time to diminish any of your premenstrual stress.

To a certain extent, exercise also reduces the appetite. For example, after a vigorous run, or perhaps a session of aerobics, you don't necessarily feel ravenously hungry as you might at the end of a hard day at work. In comparison, the pressures of a normal day's activities increase the outpouring of blood glucose which, in turn, often results in hypoglycemia and an increase in appetite. Exercise, on the other hand, causes the body to produce the glucose that it needs for its reserves of glycogen while, at the same time, mobilizing some of its fat. Hence, the blood level of glucose never actually becomes significantly elevated, so the level of insulin is only moderate, while the blood level of glucose remains fairly constant and normal. Thus, when you finish a period of exercise, you're not starving to death, but feeling "up" and full of natural energy. Another real plus for exercise is it's effect on our metabolism. Many studies show that exercise in fact speeds up our metabolic rate for several hours after a strenuous exercise period, causing us to burn calories more quickly. This means you can either exercise and eat more if you wish to remain at your present weight, or exercise and eat the same and either lose weight or stop gaining depending upon your particular diet and body type. With a regular exercise program you'll not only feel better, you'll look better too.

As you can see, the benefits of exercise are numerous and can make a difference in your PMS and your life.

The Superwoman Syndrome

Recently a TV talk show host announced, "Superwoman is dead; she died of exhaustion" and it occurred to me how true this really is for so many women in the 80's. Today's woman tries to be everything to everybody, except perhaps herself. Women are generally the primary care-givers in a family. Their numerous roles as wife, mother, businesswoman, financial planner, etc. can cause both physical and emotional stress, as well as a redefinition of self-image. I believe it's time women began to take a hard look at the quality of their lives. The first step for women is to start taking care of themselves. I'm not talking about neglecting family members or business commitments. On the contrary, women whose own needs are met will be better able to meet the needs of others. I know from personal experience that if I feel good, I can accomplish much more and have a better attitude about those accomplishments.

The Premenstrual Solution is a complete program that can defeat PMS forever, as well as increase well-being and general health. In order to maximize these positive effects, you must first take a hard look at your life. This is not always an easy thing to do, especially when a woman is under that PMS dark cloud. The best time to take stock, and begin to plan ahead is after the period, when things tend to look better.

Initially it is important to look at the areas in your life that you are happy with, and then begin to assess the areas that need a little work. Above all, be practical. Don't take on more than you can handle when you are premenstrual. I know I often felt I needed to prove I was capable of being the best mother, worker, spouse, etc. during my worst PMS. I would volunteer to bake cookies for school, cook dinners for company, work extra hours for co-workers, all in an attempt to prove to myself I was not suffering from PMS—I was a super-woman, and frankly I almost did die of exhaustion! For me, this behavior was clearly denial and only served to increase my symptoms and trigger a severe PMS crisis.

Eventually, I began to plan ahead to make life a little easier on myself before my periods. If my daughter needed cookies for school and I was premenstrual, I bought them. When my PMS symptoms were severe, I served my family a simple dinner or they prepared it themselves rather than risk a gourmet meal thrown at them in a PMS rage! When it was impossible for me to plan ahead, and I found myself falling down that PMS dark hole, I learned to take a deep breath and ask for help. In the beginning, it was difficult to admit I needed help; my style had always been to scream accusations. Nor do I think I am atypical. Now I emphatically believe that it is critical to enlist other family members when you are feeling free of PMS, so that they can be a source of help and support when you are not

Begin to take care of yourself by first making a commitment to this entire program. Plan a program of regular stress reduction such as biofeedback, yoga, hypnosis or whatever you find most relaxing. If you are not familiar with these different techniques, take responsibility for your well-being and become familiar with them. I personally use biofeedback and hypnosis as well as relaxation tapes, and I find them invaluable tools in the treatment of PMS. Anthony Mangan of Weldon Associates has several tapes on sleep and relaxation that I highly recommend to women. These tapes are excellent and can help immensely with your stress. It is important to stick to a good, nutritious diet which will add to your body's energy and vitality. Sleep enough hours to give your body adequate time to rejuvenate. It is also critical that women suffering from PMS maintain a regular schedule of taking their vitamins and minerals and most important, their tryptophan. I will discuss my recommendations for dosage in the next chapter. Women need to make time for themselves during each day, time to do something fun and relaxing such as watching T.V., reading, sewing, etc. Women also need to look at their work environment and assess the impact of this environment on their lives. It is important to attempt to find work that is satisfying and fulfilling. While this may not always be possible, the first step in developing a lifestyle that is satisfying is to recognize the areas that need work and to begin to slowly make changes in those areas. As I mentioned earlier, exercise is also a very good form of stress reduction when used to your advantage. Be realistic and patient, and realize that change takes time. Whatever you do, don't give up; this program really does work. Which brings me to . . .

Attitude

There have been numerous books written on the effects of a positive attitude on diseases such as cancer. A positive attitude is also a key ingredient in The Premenstrual Solution. Begin to visualize what it would be like to live a life free of PMS. I can tell you from personal experience that it is everything I had imagined and more. In many ways I feel that I have actually been released from death row. This book can give a woman the tools to build a life free of PMS, but she, *and only she,* can make the program work for her. PMS sufferers must take ownership of their disease and responsibility for eliminating it. This is a critical step and often a difficult one, but it can make a real difference between success and failure. I can't make you better, I can give you my knowledge and experience which you can choose to use or not use. This is your disease. Many of my patients find it difficult to accept the fact that they have a disease and that this is the treatment for that disease, not the cure. This treatment is ongoing, but it can result in a life *free* of PMS.

Initially I recommend that women chart their symptoms for a month or two to assess the premenstrual pattern. After this initial charting period, I then recommend that they throw these charts away and begin to keep a chart of positive events of the day. At the beginning of any process it is important to acknowledge whatever accomplishments have been made. Before going to sleep at night, and in the morning upon waking, I recommend that my patients do positive affirmations, such as "I'm okay," "I'm going to feel good tomorrow," "I'm going to get a good night's sleep," "I'm feeling better," etc. It is important to recognize the effect of negative thoughts on the unconscious, especially in combination with sleep deprivation. Brainwashing techniques often rely on sleep deprivation followed by the introduction of negative information. Women with PMS often "brainwash" themselves. While in a sleep-deprived state, they tell themselves over and over again that they don't feel well, that they are worthless, etc., instilling negative images on their subconscious. It's time to change all that and start feeding POSITIVE information to the brain.

Begin to listen to positive tapes such as the ones I recommended earlier. Try to surround yourself with positive people. If that isn't always possible, then try not to dwell on the negative. Buy some adhesive dots found in any stationery store and place them in strategic locations around the house, such as the mirror, refrigerator, etc. when you see one of these colored dots do a body check to assess your stress level. Is your neck tight? Are you feeling anxious? If the answer is yes, stop for a moment and take a few deep breaths, the kind that make your abdomen expand, and think, "relax." It really does work.

Finally, network with other women. There are millions of women like you who have similar symptoms and who can be a source of support. By talking and eventually laughing about this disease you can not only help yourself but other women as well.

All of these suggestions will help increase your neuroserotonin by decreasing your stress level. This increase in serotonin will then, in turn, increase the quantity and quality of your sleep, which will make you feel better, and get you off the PMS merry-go-round. Give yourself a little time. It can work for you; it has for me and for hundreds of other women as well.

STRESS REDUCTION AND ATTITUDE are critical to leading a life free of PMS. Here are some stress and attitude do's and don't's to help you eliminate symptoms forever.

STRESS/ ATTITUDE DO's

Do some form of regular stress reduction.

Do experiment with different forms of stress reduction to find one that you like.

Do obtain and regularly listen to the sleep tape by Anthony Mangan of Weldon and Associates designed for this program.

Do regular body checks to assess your level of stress.

Do place adhesive dots around your house to remind you to do these regular body checks.

Do diaphragmatic deep breathing—deep breaths that actually make your abdomen expand.

Do write positive affirmations daily.

Do mental positive affirmations daily.

Do decide to be happy and free of PMS forever.

Do learn to say no when you mean no.

Do take ownership of your own wellness.

Do decide that you are the one and only person who can eliminate your PMS forever.

Do share your PMS experience with other women, but do it in a positive, helpful and healing way.

Do learn to laugh and play daily.

Do plan ahead to decrease stress on known difficult
days.

Do believe that this will work for you.

STRESS/
ATTITUDE DON'T's

Don't be a superwoman.

Don't be afraid to try stress reduction techniques.

Don't over extend.

Don't make negative statements either verbally or mentally about yourself or your PMS.

Don't feel guilty; guilt will only intensify negative self
feelings and inhibit your recovery.

Don't apologize for your disease.

Don't be afraid to share your feelings with family members and friends.

Don't try to surpass your physical limitations.

Don't continue to take on more than you can handle.

Don't stop using these techniques when you start to
feel better.

Don't give up, this really works!

Case History
Number Five

The Story of Chuck

Chuck is a 34 year-old male who was referred to me by his wife. She had been a patient of mine earlier, and after I treated her successfully for her own PMS symptoms, it occurred to her that since her husband had been experiencing so many of the same psychological symptoms, perhaps my treatment program would also work for him.

In any case, by the time he came to me, Chuck had reached such a point of desperation, he told me, "Right now I'm ready to try any treatment you've got as long as it's not a sex change." When I assured him I had no such drastic tampering in mind for him, he relaxed.

Chuck had been seeing a rather costly psychiatrist for more than a year, but could no longer afford to continue those visits. Interestingly enough, I found that Chuck had had a history of nightly bedwetting as a child, which continued until puberty, but his wife had not. He held down a stressful job in electronics, and the fact that he had worked the night shift for many years had only added to that stress. He had been experiencing intermittent periods of rage and temper tantrums. He was also suffering from recurring migraine headaches, as well as violent fits of anger that often had him punching his fist through doors, after which he would dash out of the house in a screaming fury, then get in the car and drive away.

He told me his major fear during these episodes was that he would turn these feelings of rage and violence against his family. Rather than run the risk of beating his wife or his children, he usually ended up running off for a long drive until the mood passed. While she was having her own PMS problems, his wife felt that she might be the cause of his erratic mood swings. It wasn't until her own health vastly improved that she realized her husband had his own special problems. It reached the point where she could never predict when Chuck would have another of his outbursts; nor could he, as it turned out. At least she always knew what time of the month she could expect to feel lousy and, in a way, could prepare herself for the worst. But with Chuck, these moods would sometimes hit him as frequently as two or three times a week.

His psychiatrist tried him on antidepressants for a time, but though he would experience some initial relief, it would never last. I realized very quickly that it was this man's bad sleeping environment that was causing most of his problems. The fact that he was obliged to sleep days gave him a schedule that was exactly the reverse of everyone else's in the house. He complained of awakening from a day's sleep feeling even more "muddle-headed" than when he went to bed. There would be a lot of light in his room while he slept, and since his wife also worked, she wasn't there to greet their two noisy children when they came home from school. They would often run into his bedroom, demanding that he play with them. This would cause him to scare them away with the kind of temper tantrum that, again, had him worried he might someday hurt them.

Finally, after his wife's symptoms had improved with my treatment, she suggested that Chuck make an appointment with me. She gave him my name, then added, "She's a licensed Physicians Assistant, Chuck, and a real specialist."

"You think that's what I really need—to see a woman?" he had asked. "Don't tell me she's another marriage counselor."

"Not at all. Actually, she's a PMS specialist."

"PMS?" he said, gaping at her. "I don't believe it. You want me to see an expert on female problems?"

"It's worth a try, Chuck. And it's all so simple. This treatment doesn't involve anything but taking a perfectly harmless food supplement three or four times a day. No hard-core drugs, no hormone shots, nothing like that."

Finally, he agreed to make an appointment, though he first made his wife swear she would never mention this to any of their friends. In particular, he feared that if any of the guys at the plant heard about this, he would never live it down.

However, when he finally came to see me, he did not wear a disguise, nor did he use an assumed name. In fact, when he got over the novelty of exactly what my specialty was, he was very frank and open about discussing his symptoms. "But before we start," he said, "there's one thing you've got to know. I mean, I can remember some of the complaints my wife used to have when she was going through her bad times. So, right off, I want you to know I'm not feeling any breast tenderness, or water retention."

Once all that was squared away, I started him on my Tryptophan Treatment Program, and after only a month or so, he began to feel a steady improvement. He had told me that his stressful symptoms were at their worst whenever his sleep had been disrupted. Hence, as an adjunct to tryptophan, I advised him to get used to wearing a sleep mask and ear-plugs for as long as he was obliged to sleep days. Together with the Tryptophan Treatment Program these suggestions worked like a charm. And when his wife arranged it so the kids wouldn't be on hand while their father was asleep, the whole household was well on the way to total recovery. After about six months, Chuck was feeling so much better, he didn't hesitate to recommend me and my treatment plan to several of his friends, all of them male.

9

The Tryptophan Treatment Program

The Solution, at Long Last

BEFORE YOU START this program, it is important that you see your practitioner and have a thorough physical examination, which should include pelvic exam, papsmear, breast exam, and screening blood work. This blood work should include a complete blood count, blood chemistry, thyroid function tests and, if you are close to menopause, a follical stimulating hormone level to asses if some of your symptoms are a result of early or normal menopause. It is important to make sure symptoms are a result of PMS and not another underlying disease such as anemia.

It is important that women who are pregnant, or who are planning to become pregnant immediately, *not* take tryptophan. If you should become pregnant while taking tryptophan, stop taking it and talk with your practioner. Women who are taking antidepressants or MAO inhibitors should not take tryptophan before talking with their practitioners. Perhaps they can taper off these medications and start tryptophan. These decisions, however, should be made by a professional.

Tryptophan is currently classified by the FDA as a food supplement and can be obtained over the counter at most health food stores and supermarkets. I feel strongly that the dosages recommend in this book are safe. As previously discussed in this text, tryptophan is found in many foods that you consume daily. However, because foods contain many different amino acids other than tryptophan alone, these amino acids all have to compete to cross into the brain. This competition actually decreases the amount of tryptophan that gets into the brain. Because of the problems with getting tryptophan across the blood brain barrier, I recommend that it be taken in tablet form as opposed to only eating foods high in tryptophan. It has been available in tablet form for a number of years. As a food supplement, it has been found to be safe and effective by the FDA; however, a recent study, which you may have read about, stated that when rats were given very high doses of tryptophan they developed changes in their livers. The adult equivalent to these dosages are much higher than anyone would ever take. After doing liver function tests on my patients and myself, I have found no such effect in the small dosages I recommend nor have there been any studies to substantiate these findings in humans. But, be safe and have regular examinations by your practitioner.

It has been my experience that a patient should begin by taking 500 mg. of tryptophan three times per day.

One tablet should be taken midmorning, one midafternoon, and one midevening on an empty stomach with a carbohydrate such as fruit juice, whole wheat crackers, fruit or a fructose based soft drink. When I say an empty stomach, I mean either two hours after a meal or one hour before a meal. *DO NOT TAKE TRYPTOPHAN WITH PROTEIN.* It will not hurt you if you take it with a protein; however, it will not work nearly as effectively. If you find you can't fit in a dosage because of your particular meal schedule, rather than miss a dosage altogether, take the tryptophan. However, realize that it does not work as well when taken with protein. This dosage should then be increased to four or five tablets a day approximately two or three days before ovulation. Many of my patients do well on a three/four regimen; however, some require as many as six in the second half of their cycle. Dosages do not always seem to correlate with severity of symptoms. I would, therefore, suggest you start with a three/four routine and adjust up accordingly. Keeping in mind that this will not work if you are not getting adequate sleep.

The first week you are taking tryptophan you will probably notice an increase in dreaming, for many women this has been quite dramatic. Although I thought I had been dreaming prior to starting on the tryptophan, I found, as have most of my patients, that after I started the program the dreaming was in color and quite vivid, not an unpleasant experience. However, initially I did feel that I was not sleeping quite as soundly. This change in the sleep pattern is REM rebound, i.e., we are actually catching up on REM sleep. This REM rebound will last only a few days, so don't worry about it. Although you may feel that you are not sleeping as well the first week on the program, you will probably notice that you feel slightly more rested upon awakening, assuming you are sleeping an adequate amount.

Because the conversion of serotonin to melatonin is controlled by our perception of light and dark, tryptophan should not make you sleepy during the day. When you close your eyes at night you will become drowsy and fall asleep. If you have had problems with insomnia give this program a little time, and it will work for you, too.

I can't emphasize enough the importance of sleep to the elimination of the emotional symptoms of PMS. Without adequate amounts of sleep the symptoms simply will not go away. I feel I need a minimum of eight hours during my postmenstrual phase and somewhere between nine and ten hours when I am premenstrual. This varies from woman to woman. I know it may sound like a lot of sleep, but the rewards far out number the sacrifices for me and my family, friends, co-workers, and even strangers. Find that critical number of hours that will make the difference for you and then stick with it.

As described in the previous chapter, be aware of the value of a regular program of stress reduction. The biofeedback sleep tape developed by Anthony Mangan for this program helps promote a better quality of sleep by teaching the subconscious how to better utilize tryptophan in the production of serotonin. I would recommend that you take time to lie down and listen to this tape in a quiet, dark room on a daily basis the first month or two of the program, and then, perhaps, the two weeks prior to your period in subsequent months.

ESPECIALLY FOR WOMEN

Especially for women is part of the Tryptophan Treatment Program designed to help eliminate your PMS. This program contains 1-Tryptophan and a multivitamin and multimineral that I have specifically formulated after years of researching this problem in women. I continue to get reports from my patients telling me how much better they feel on this product. It is specially coated to help make it easy to swallow and priced to make it affordable.

* Easy to swallow because it is coated

* Priced to make it affordable

* Specifically formulated for the needs of women with PMS

* Multivitamin/multimineral contains 180 tablets per bottle

* 1-Tryptophane contains 150 tablets per bottle

* Order form and other information are located in the back of the book

Vitamin/Mineral Chart

<u>SIX TABLETS PROVIDE:</u>

BETA CAROTENE (Vit. A Equivalent) . . . 15,000 I.U.
VITAMIN A (Palmitate-Water
    Dispersible) . . . . 5,000 I.U.
VITAMIN C (Corn Free-Ascorbic Acid) . . . 1,200 mg
VITAMIN D-3 (Cholecalciferol) . . . . 200 I.U.
VITAMIN E (d-Alpha Tocopherol
    Succinate) . . . . 200 I.U.
BOIFLAVONOIDS (25% Hesperidin
    content) . . . . 250 mg

VITAMIN B-1 . . . . 100 mg
VITAMIN B-2 . . . . 100 mg
NIACINAMIDE . . . . 100 mg
PANTOTHENIC ACID . . . . 150 mg
VITAMIN B-6 . . . . 150 mg
VITAMIN B-12 (on ion exchange resin) . . . . 125 mcg
BIOTIN . . . . 30 mcg
FOLIC ACID . . . . 800 mcg
CHOLINE . . . . 300 mg

CALCIUM (Aspartate Complex) . . . . 500 mg
MAGNESIUM (Aspartate Complex) . . . . 500 mg
POTASSIUM (Chloride) . . . . 95 mg
IRON (Ferronyl™-carbonyl iron) . . . . 25 mg
COPPER (Amino Acid Chelate) . . . . 2 mg
ZINC (Amino Acid Chelate) . . . . 30 mg
MANGANESE (Amino Acid Chelate)* . . . . . . 20 mg
BORON (Amino Acid Chelate)* . . . . 3 mg
IODINE (Kelp) . . . . 200 mcg

CHROMIUM (Amino Acid Chelate)* . . . . 500 mcg
SELENIUM (Amino Acid Chelate)* . . . . 100 mcg
MOLYBDENUM (Amino Acid Chelate)* . . . . . 50 mcg
VANADIUM (Amino Acid Chelate)* . . . . 25 mcg

Other Ingredients (Descending order of weight)

PABA (Para Amino   Pancreatin (High Lipase)
  Benzoic Acid)   Inositol
Rutin

*CHELATES ARE ALL YEAST & SOYA FREE (Rice
  Protein Chelates)

Directions:

As a dietary supplement suggested use 2 tablets 3
times per day with meals or as suggested by your
physician.

This promotes relaxation as well as helps us to better utilize serotonin. After nearly two years of being symptom-free I still continue to listen to sleep tapes and biofeedback tapes to help promote my own well being, and it works.

As previously discussed in the chapter on nutrition, it is not necessary to drastically modify your diet in an attempt to stop your PMS. The changes are really simple and easy to follow. AVOID ARTIFICIAL SWEETENERS AT ALL COSTS, PARTICULARLY THOSE CONTAINING PHENYLALININE. Phenylalinine blocks tryptophan from crossing the blood brain barrier and actually magnifies the symptoms. Use moderation and good sense when using caffeine, alcohol and sugar. This does not mean that you can never eat or drink foods which contain these ingredients. What it does mean is that you should be particularly careful when you are premenstrual. It is also important for your good health to increase your consumption of complex carbohydrates, vegetables and fruits, and to decrease your consumption of fat. Again, moderation is the key; enjoy your life, but consider your overall health.

If you are currently taking sleeping pills, tranquilizers, antidepressants, antihistamines or other PMS formulations such as progesterone or evening primrose, I would suggest you speak with your practitioner about discontinuing these medications. It has been my experience that this program is not as effective when used in combination with other therapies such as progesterone. For many women, it is a difficult step to consider discontinuing the use of progesterone or other remedies that may be giving them some marginal relief. However, after a month or two on my program my patients without exception have been thankful for my insistence on a drug free approach to PMS.

The importance of exercise in a program of good health is essential, and is also very important to the PMS woman. This exercise, as previously described should be done if possible in the afternoon, or, if not, in the morning. Evening exercise should be avoided as it decreases REM sleep. Although I feel exercise is very important, it is often the final step in the PMS program and one that took me, personally, almost a year of being symptom-free to become committed to. Initially, I began very slowly, and now I weighttrain approximately two hours per day, six afternoons a week, and I love the way I feel and the way my body is beginning to look. Start a program of exercise slowly and don't give up. It is important that your PMS be somewhat better before you start a rigorous program.

This program has literally changed my life. I no longer suffer from fatigue. When I awaken in the morning I feel refreshed and rested, ready to begin a new day. I feel younger and more vital than I have in more than ten years and this feeling continues all month long. I no longer have to consciously remember to follow the program as outlined in this book, because it has become second nature to me. The positive results are too good for me to deviate from my tried and true routine. I no longer feel irritable before my periods. I have no rage attacks or depression. I can't tell you the last time I cried over something insignificant. The biggest change is that I feel happy and content most of the time. My relationships with my husband and daughter have improved considerably, and they no longer fear my PMS because it is finally and permanently under control. I have done this for myself, and I have given you the opportunity to do it for yourself as well. It really is up to you.

Be patient. Give this program a little time. You will probably begin to notice an improvement in your fatigue initially. This improvement will probably begin anywhere from a week to a month, depending on the amount of sleep you are getting. Emotional symptoms will begin to slowly dissipate over the first three months of this program. You may notice at first that you hesitate prior to a rage attack, or that your depression is improving. Look at these changes with a positive attitude and feel hopeful. It's OK to be hopeful; you won't be disappointed. Physical symptoms such as breast tenderness and bloating may take as long as six months. They will eventually go away as well. Your symptoms will continue to improve for six months to a year at which time you should stabalize. REMEMBER, THE NUMBER OF HOURS YOU SLEEP IS WHAT MAKES THE DIFFERENCE.

On a Note of Conclusion

Some Last-Minute Tips

AFTER BEING ON THIS PROGRAM, PMS patients should experience only the more normal feelings healthy women get during their period. Women who do not have PMS go through the usual organic symptoms, but they don't consider it a special problem.

Perhaps a day or two before their period they might feel a little more tired than usual, but they never feel out of control and suffer no cyclic depression or rage. Thus, this time of the month passes, leaving no real debilitating effects on them. These are the kind of results we are aiming for.

Ironically, many women who do *not* have PMS can often pose a serious challenge for PMS victims. These women are the most difficult to convince there *is* such a problem as PMS, simply because they've never had such symptoms themselves. These are the women who resent the recent media attention being given to PMS.

Consequently, they might say, "Oh, that's all in their minds!" thereby dismissing PMS sufferers as being neurotic, unstable or psychosomatic. Because they don't have these symptoms, they lack the ability to empathize with someone who does.

For the most part, these are contemporary women who may feel they're having enough conflicts trying to compete with men in the work-place without introducing the distinctly female and humiliating possibility of PMS.

However, criticism and resistance to PMS as a legitimate disease comes from other sectors of our society as well. For example, I spoke to one lady in her late fifties who had been a housewife and mother all her life.

She had this to say: "Now in my day, we didn't make such a silly fuss about things like that. This is a private, intimate subject, to be kept between you and the Lord. Today's females are so pampered and self-indulgent, they stubbornly refuse to resign themselves to a problem God has designed for all of us to bear in silence." Here was a women who obviously never had a problem with PMS. And since nobody spoke about this subject in "her day," there was really no way for her to know how many women were suffering a great deal more than she was. In essence, her reaction to PMS is analogous to that of someone who doesn't have diabetes telling a diabetes patient, "Oh, just go ahead and eat the chocolate cake and stop worrying. It never bothers *me!*"

The acceptance of PMS as a reality for *some* women is a vital issue for *all* women and men too, for that matter. Women must shed the fear that public knowledge of PMS might disqualify them from the marketplace or destroy their credibility in personal relationships. Suffering in silence is not the answer and never has been. On the contrary, it's only by confronting the reality of PMS and publicizing it in the media that PMS victims can at last find out what's causing their symptoms and abolish them. Thus, it's more information we need, not more secrecy. Once PMS is confronted with honesty and compassion, we will be able to talk about it as something that *used* to bother us, but which is no longer a problem.

I urge my patients to involve their families in their treatment program and not shroud their problem in mystery. PMS requires acceptance and understanding especially from those who are closest to us. The patient needs to recognize this and ask for cooperation on bad days and frankly tell both husband and children exactly how they can help ease the tension. Support and cooperation from families is indispensible for the PMS patient.

The trouble with many women, however, is that they will force themselves to do whatever's necessary without even mentioning how they feel, possibly because of guilt about having the problem in the first place, or perhaps out of a sense of failure in not living up to expectations about their "role" in the family. Women must get over the feeling that they are "disqualifying" themselves whenever they mention PMS related symptoms, and remember that many other menstruating women experience this problem to one degree or another, and that it is nothing to be ashamed of.

Although you will feel vast improvements after a few months of my Tryptophan Treatment Program, you aren't going to remain in a state of gleeful joy for the rest of your life. You will still have days when you may feel normal depression, though probably for reasons other than being premenstrual. This treatment will, however, take away those cyclic feelings of tension, rage and despair.

A word of caution: although I noticed improvements after being on the program only a week or two, I found that it took my family several months to be convinced. Initially, I don't think my family really believed my condition had improved. I now feel sure this is because they had become as programmed as I was to expect certain behavior at that time of the month. As a result, I guess they wanted to reserve judgment, lest I revert to the same old mood-swings the next time around. Consequently, even after my condition improved to the point where I was no longer being testy or moody during my cycle, all I'd have to do is get normally irritable for a good reason, and my husband might say, "it must be that time of the month again." I was, in fact, cured a lot faster than my family, since there was no medication that would change their way of relating to me overnight. I realized what was happening, however, and was patient.

Women in this program must exercise patience as they wait for the results. Ideally, a woman should be on the treatment program for at least three to six months to begin to experience physical and emotional improvements in their PMS. As might be expected, the emotional symptoms are the first to be alleviated, while such physical symptoms as breast tenderness and bloating take longer. The only reports of bad results I have gotten are from those impatient souls who don't stay with the program long enough, some of them giving it only a two or three days' trial. I now urge my patients not to expect to notice any improvements that quickly. After all, isn't it a little unrealistic to expect instant relief from a problem that's been driving you up the wall ever since puberty?

It is also important to reemphasize that the key to relieving these PMS symptoms is *normal sleep*. It's true that tryptophan helps you to sleep, but sleep is the solution!

I foresee a time in the not too distant future when PMS will take its place in history with other diseases like the black plague and diptheria as an illness of the past. But before that happens, women will have to take the initiative by casting off the stigma attached to PMS. How? By confronting the disease and taking personal responsibility for defeating it.

Such an assertive action requires honesty with self and others—a willingness to confront one's own areas of vulnerability, to dismiss outdated self-images, to see clearly the areas in one's personal and professional life that reflect the disease, and to ask for help when appropriate. Women must not only be willing to admit that there is a problem, they must also have a clear conviction that there is a solution, and finally, they must have faith in themselves and their ability to implement it.

Despite the magnitude of the challenge, there are many women like myself who have already pursued the process and radically changed their lives and the lives of those around them. The proof that PMS can be controlled is unmistakable. The beauty of the Premenstrual Solution is that it is easily accessible and merely requires perseverance and commitment—a small price to pay for a new lease on life.

Perhaps the most satisfying aspect of my work has

been watching my patients take control of their lives once again. I have seen how their personal revolution against the destructive forces of PMS translates into physical well being, increased self-esteem, personal growth and happiness, family harmony and even career advancement. The time has come for both men and women to set aside old taboos, misconceptions, personal grievances and to lend their support to the PMS revolution. The goal is in sight. All that remains is to reach out for it.

References

1) Brush MG, Watson SJ, Horrobin DF, Phil D, Manku MS. *Abnormal Essential Fatty Acid Levels in Plasma of Women with Premenstrual Syndrome.* **American Journal of Obstetrics and Gynecology.** October 15, 1984; pp. 383–366.

2) Reid RL, Yen SSC. *Premenstrual Syndrome.* **American Journal of Obstetrics and Gynecology.** January, 1981; pp. 139, 85–104.

3) Muse KN, Cetel NS, Futterman LA, Yen SSC. *The Premenstrual Syndrome: Effects of "Medical Ovariectomy."* **New England Journal of Medicine.** 1984; pp. 311, 1345–1349.

4) Munoz RA. *Postpartum Psychosis as a Discrete Entity.* **Journal of Clinical Psychiatry.** 46:5. May, 1985; pp. 182–184.

5) Steege JF, Stout AL, Rupp SL. *Relationships Among Premenstrual Symptoms and Menstrual Cycle Characteristics.* **Obstetrics and Gynecology.** 65:3. March, 1985; pp. 398–402.

6) Sheehan DY, Carr DB, Fishman SM, Walsh MM, Peltier-Saxe D. *Lactate Infusion in Anxiety Research: Its Evolution and Practice.* **Journal of Clinical Psychiatry.** 46:5. May, 1985; pp. 158–165.

7) Montgomery SA. *Development of New Treatments for Depression.* **Journal of Clinical Psychiatry.** 46:3. Section 2. March, 1985; pp. 3–6.

8) Rickels K, Feighner JP, Smith WT. *Alprazolam, Amitriptyline, Doxepin, and Placebo in the Treatment of Depression.* **Archive of General Psychology.** Volume 42. February, 1985; pp. 134–140.

9) Wurtman RJ. *The Ultimate Head Waiter: How the Brain Controls Diet.* **Technology Review.** July, 1974; pp. 42, 51.

10) Fellman B. *A Clockwork Gland.* **Science.** May, 1985; pp. 77–81.

11) Halbreich U, Endicott J, Nee J. *Premenstrual Depressive Changes: Value of Differentiation.* **Archive of General Psychology.** Volume 40. May, 1983; pp. 535–542.

12) DeLaFuente JR, Rosenbaum AH. *Prolactin in Psychiatry.* **American Journal Of Psychology.** 138:9. September, 1981; pp. 1154–1158.

13) Lemberger L, Bergstrom RF, Wolen RL, Farid NA, Enas GG, Aronoff GR. *Fluoxetine: Clinical Pharmacology and Physiologic Disposition.* **Journal of Clinical Physology.** 46:3. Section 2. March, 1985; pp. 14–19.

14) Stark P, Fuller RW, Wong DT. *The Pharmacologic Profile of Fluoxetine.* **Journal of Clinical Psychology.** 46:3. Section 2. March, 1985; pp. 7–12.

15)   Taylor DL, Mather RJ, Ho BT, Weinman ML. *Serotonin Levels and Platelet Uptake During Premenstrual Tension.* **Neuropsychobiology.** 1984; pp. 16–18.

16)   Bancroft J, Backstrom T. *Premenstrual Syndrome (Review).* **Clinical Endocrinology.** 1985; pp. 22, 313–336.

17)   Abraham S. *Premenstrual or Postmenstrual Syndrome?* **The Medical Journal of Australia.** September, 1984; pp. 327–328.

18)   Rausch JL, Janowsky DS, Risch SC, Judd LL, Huey LY. *Hormonal and Neurotransmitter Hypotheses of Premenstrual Tension (Review).* **Psychopharmacology Bulletin.** 18:4. October, 1982; pp. 26–34.

19)   Harrison W, Lharge L, Endicott J. *Treatment of Premenstrual Symptoms.* **General Hospital Psychology.** 1985; pp. 54–65.

20)   Biegon A, Reches A, Snyder S, McEwan BS. *Serotonergic and Noradrenergic Receptors in the Rat Brain: Modulation by Chronic Exposure to Ovarian Hormones.* **Life Sciences.** Volume 32. 1983; pp. 2015–2021.

21)   Brelje M. *PMS: The Total Picture.* **Colorado Medicine.** July, 1984; pp. 165–166.

22)   Deleon-Jones FA, Val E, Herts C. *MHPG Excretion and Lithium Treatment During Premenstrual Tension Syndrome: A Case Report.* **American Journal of Psychiatry.** 139:7. July, 1982; pp. 950–951.

23) Blume E. *Premenstrual Syndromes, Depression Linked.* **Journal of the American Medical Association.** 249:21. June, 1983; pp. 2864–2866.

24) Friedman RC, Hurt SW, Clarkin J, Corn R, Aronoff MS. *Sexual Histories and Premenstrual Affective Syndrome in Psychiatric Inpatients.* **American Journal of Psychology.** 139:11. 1982; pp. 1484–1486.

25) O'Brien P, Selby C, Symonds EM. *Progesterone, Fluid and Electrolytes in Premenstrual Syndrome.* **British Medical Journal.** May, 1980; pp. 1161–1162.

25) O'Brien P. *The Premenstrual Syndrome: A Review of the Present Status of Therapy.* **Drugs 24.** 1982; pp. 140–151.

26) Lauersen NH, Graves ZR. *A New Approach to Premenstrual Syndrome.* **The Female Patient.** Volume 8. April, 1983; pp. 41–52.

27) Ylostalo P, Kauppila A, Puolakka J, Ronnberg L, Janne O. *Bromocriptine and Norethisterone in the Treatment of Premenstrual Syndrome.* **Obstetrics and Gynecology.** 59:3. March, 1982; pp. 292–297.

28) Elsner CW, Buster JE, Schindler RA, Nessim SA, Abraham GE. *Bromocriptine in the Treatment of Premenstrual Tension Syndrome.* **Obstetrics and Gynecology.** 56:6. December, 1980; pp. 723–725.

29) Freeman EW, Sondheimer S, Weinbaum PJ, Rickels K. *Evaluating Premenstrual Symptoms in Medical Practice.* **Obstetrics and Gynecology.** 65:4. April, 1985; pp. 500–505.

30) Price WA, Giannini AJ. *The Use of Clonidine in Premenstrual Tension Syndrome.* **Journal of Clinical Pharmacology.** 1984; pp. 24, 463–465.

31) Brunetti LL, Taff ML. *The Premenstrual Syndrome.* **The American Journal of Forensic Medicine and Pathology.** 5:3. September, 1984; pp. 265–268.

32) Lyon KE, Lyon MA. *The Premenstrual Syndrome: A Survey of Current Treatment Practices.* **The Journal of Reproductive Medicine.** 29:10. October, 1984; pp. 705–711.

33) O'Brien P. *The Premenstrual Syndrome: A Review.* **The Journal of Reproductive Medicine.** 30:2. February, 1985; pp. 113–126.

34) London RS, Sundaram G, Manimekalai S, Murphy L, Raynolds M, Goldstein P. *The Effect of Alpha-Tocopherol on Premenstrual Symptomatology: A Double-Blind Study, Endocrine Correlates.* **Journal of the American College of Nutrition 3.** February, 1984; pp. 351–356.

35) Giannini AJ, Price WA, Loiselle RH. *B-Endorphin Withdrawal: A Possible Cause of Premenstrual Tension Syndrome.* **International Journal of Psychophysiology 1.** 1984; pp. 341–343.

36) Faratian H, Johnson IR, Prescott P. *Premenstrual Syndrome: Weight, Abdominal Swelling, and Perceived Body Image.* **American Journal of Obstetrics and Gynecology.** September, 1984; pp. 200–204.

37) Canty AP. *Can Aerobic Exercise Relieve the Symptoms of Premenstrual Syndrome (PMS)?* **JOSH.** 54:10. November, 1984; pp.410–411.

38) Adams W, Rose P, Foldard, Wynn V, Seed M, Strong R. *Effect of Pyridoxine Hydrochloride (Vitamin B6) Upon Depression Associated with Oral Contraceptives.* **The Lancet.** April, 1973; pp. 897–903.

39) Wintrobe, Thorn, Adams, Brainwald, Isselbueber, Petersdorf. **Harrison's Principles of Internal Medicine.** 7th Edition. pp. 125–130; 427–430.

40) Watts JF, Butt WR, Edwards, Logan R, Holder G. *Hormonal Studies in Women with Premenstrual Tension.* **British Journal of Obstetrics and Gynecology.** Volume 92. March, 1985; pp. 247–255.

41) Williams, Robert H. **Textbook of Endocrinology.** W B Saunders Company.

42) Ford N. **Good Night. The Easy and Natural Way to Sleep the Whole Night Through.** 1983.

43) Weideger P. **Menstruation and Menopause: The Physiology and Psychology, the Myth and the Reality.** 1976.

INFORMATION/ORDER FORM

☐ 1-tryptophane (150 tablets per bottle) $24.95

☐ Multivitamin/multimineral (180 tablets per bottle) $14.95

☐ The Pre-Menstrual Solution Book $14.95

☐ Information regarding seminars and lectures by Jo Ann Cutler Friedrich, P.A.

Please add $3.00 for shipping and handling of each order and make check payable to Arrow Press.

NAME _____

ADDRESS _____

_____

TO: ARROW PRESS, INC.
     1228 Lincoln Avenue, Suite 103
     San Jose, California 95125